The Effective Ketogenic

s

The Ultimate 5-Week Meal Plan for Sustainable Weight Loss

Chef Effect

Table of Contents

Introduction

The ketogenic diet offers this premise: eat 60-90% of your calories from fat, adapt to metabolizing fat quickly as energy, gain better appetite control and regulation, and lose weight as your body easily burns fat stores. It sounds like the complete opposite of everything we've been told about weight loss for the past few decades, but strong research backs up the science behind the ketogenic diet. As you replace most of the carbohydrates in your diet with fat, major physiological changes occur that make it easier for many people to lose weight. In most cases, they also see lower blood pressure and cholesterol and other health benefits!

This book is a complete guide to beginning the ketogenic diet. We'll explain what it is, the basics of how ketosis works, and who should and shouldn't follow this diet. We'll tell you what to eat and what to avoid, give you key advice about maximizing the effectiveness of the diet, and, best of all, provide you with over ninety delicious recipes for breakfast, lunch, dinner, and snacks. Enjoy!

What is the Ketogenic Diet?

The ketogenic diet is based on using fat, rather than carbohydrates, as the primary source of energy. The diet is designed to result in ketosis, a state in which your body produces a molecule called ketones from fat molecules that you eat. Ketones, instead of glucose, become the primary energy molecule in your body. The ketogenic diet can aid in weight loss because, as your body becomes adapted to burning fat as fuel, it draws upon body fat reserves rather than burning carbohydrates and storing excess energy as fat.

The ketogenic diet was first developed as a treatment for drug resistant epilepsy about one hundred years ago and is still used as one of the most effective treatments for a range of seizure disorders. Over time, doctors noticed that other physiological effects resulted from this diet. Potential benefits from following the ketogenic diet include weight loss, better appetite control, increased and more consistent energy levels, better insulin sensitivity, treatment of insulin-related disorders like diabetes, and fewer damaging effects from high or highly variable blood glucose levels.

The standard ketogenic diet entails extreme carbohydrate restriction, with carbohydrates accounting for 3-5% of total calories, protein supplying 7-10%, and fat supplying 85-90%. This is very hard to follow and is mostly used in clinical settings. The modified ketogenic diet offers many of the same benefits with greater flexibility. Carbohydrates supply 5-13% of calories, protein supplies 15-30%, and fat supplies 60 to 80%, with saturated fat supplying no more than 20% of total calories.

What is Ketosis?

Ketosis is a physiological state characterized by the production of *ketones* by the body and their presence in the blood. The production of these small molecules is known as *ketogenesis*. Let's break down these terms and explain what happens when you eat a ketogenic diet.

Normally, carbohydrates supply most of the energy in our diets – anywhere from 50 to 70%. All digestible carbohydrates (fiber is a non-digestible carbohydrate) are broken down into glucose, a simple sugar molecule that is then transported around the body and converted to other energy-rich molecules that cells can use to carry out the thousands of chemical reactions essential for life. A key intermediary molecule in this process is acetyl, a 2-carbon molecule. Glucose must be converted to acetyl before it can be used to supply energy; fat molecules must also be broken down to form acetyl before they can be used to supply energy.

These acetyl molecules combine with CoA to form acetyl CoA, which feeds into the Citric Acid Cycle, an essential metabolic step. Another key molecule for the Citric Acid Cycle is oxaloacetate. This can be supplied by both carbohydrates and protein, but not by fat. To summarize, our bodies need both acetyl and oxaloacetate to run the Citric Acid Cycle and convert the energy to a form that all cells can use. A diet with a mix of carbohydrates, fat, and protein will supply plenty of acetyl and plenty of oxaloacetate, but a diet very high in fat and very low in carbohydrates will supply a lot of acetyl and very little oxaloacetate.

This, the imbalance of acetyl and oxaloacetate in the liver, is the essential condition for ketosis. When this occurs, the body must use a different type of reaction to produce useful energy. The excess acetyl from fat is converted into a type of molecule known as a ketone body, which can be used by most cells in the body for energy.

Ketosis can occur for several reasons, not just as a result of the ketogenic diet. During fasting, blood glucose is very low and the body must rely exclusively on stored fat, resulting in the same acetyl oversupply. During endurance exercise, the body also starts drawing on fat stores and converting excess acetyl to ketone bodies. In addition, ketosis can occur during uncontrolled diabetes, when insufficient insulin is produced to signal glucose uptake and cells must rely on fat instead.

Who Should Follow the Ketogenic Diet?

Most people who are young to middle-aged, relatively fit, and do not suffer from acute or chronic disease can follow the ketogenic diet without problems. If you are older than fifty, in poor physical health, or suffer from chronic diseases such as diabetes, you may be able to benefit from the ketogenic diet, but it is important to begin it only under the supervision of a doctor. Pregnant or breastfeeding women, young children, people with kidney or liver disease, and those with other serious health issues should never attempt the ketogenic diet on their own – only when directed to do so by a medical professional.

What to Eat for the Ketogenic Diet

How Much Fat, Protein, Carbohydrates, and Total Calories to Consume

While following the ketogenic diet, it is *essential* to keep track of calorie and macronutrient (fat, protein, carb) totals and percentages. Over-consuming calories on the ketogenic diet is harmful to the body and can lead to weight gain and fat accumulation in the liver. Over consuming carbohydrates and protein will prevent you from maintaining ketosis.

Consume no more calories than you burn each day, or 200-400 fewer, especially if you are trying to lose weight. Over time, the ketogenic diet usually leads to decreased appetite and caloric intake with no effort, but it may be difficult in the first few weeks to ensure that you do not over consume calories. Also keep in mind that ketogenic meals are quite calorie dense, since they are so high in fat. As a result, portions may seem small, even though they are high in calories. Below, we provide general guidelines for fat, protein, and carbohydrate intake for ketogenic diets at four caloric intake levels. If you follow the meal plan provided, you may need to reduce or increase portion sizes to meet your specific needs.

For a 2,200 calorie diet:

> Fat: 60-80%, 1,320-1,760 calories, 147-196g, no more than 40-45g saturated fat

> Protein: 15-30%, 330- 660 calories, 82.5-165g

> Carbohydrates: 5-9%, 110-200 calories, 27.5-50g

For a 2,000 calorie diet:

> Fat: 60-80%, 1,200-1,600 calories, 133-178g, no more than 40g saturated fat

> Protein: 15-30%, 300- 600 calories, 75-150g

> Carbohydrates: 5-10%, 100-200 calories, 25-50g

For a 1,800 calorie diet:

> Fat: 60-80%, 1,200-1,600 calories, 133-178g, no more than 40g saturated fat

> Protein: 15-30%, 270-540 calories, 68-135g

> Carbohydrates: 5-11%, 90-200 calories, 22.5-50g

For a 1,600 calorie diet:

> Fat: 60-80%, 1,200-1,600 calories, 133-178g, no more than 35g saturated fat

Protein: 15-30%, 240-480 calories, 60-120g

Carbohydrates: 5-12.5%, 80-200 calories, 20-50g

Fat Sources for the Ketogenic Diet

While following the ketogenic diet, you will get 70 to 85% of your daily calories from fat. This means that you will be eating *a lot* of fat. All fat is not created equal – in fact, there are dozens of different fatty acids, all with distinct physiological effects – so it's essential that you carefully assess the types you plan to include so as to create a diet that is tasty, highly conducive to ketosis, heart-healthy, and environmentally sustainable.

One of the most important types of fat to include in a ketogenic diet is medium-chain fatty acids. You can also get a large portion of your fat from monounsaturated long-chain fatty acids, found in foods like olive oil, nuts, and avocados. Omega-3 fatty acids are essential for brain health and reducing inflammation and need to be included in small quantities. In general, you will need to avoid consuming excessive amounts of saturated and omega-6 fatty acids and avoid trans fatty acids completely. Below, we'll explain more about each type of fat and what types of foods provide it.

Medium-Chain Triglycerides (MCTs)

An important type of fat to include in ketogenic diets is MCT. MCT stands for medium-chain triglyceride, a type of fat that has eight to twelve carbon atoms in its fatty acid tail. In contrast, long-chain fatty acids, which make up the vast majority of fat in our diet, have fourteen to twenty-two carbon atoms in the tail. These types of fats are processed very differently by the body. Long-chain fatty acids are absorbed from the small intestine into the lymphatic system. Along with cholesterol, they get packaged into small spheres known as chylomicrons and circulate throughout the body. As a result, there are many opportunities for these circulating long-chain fatty acids to be taken in by adipose cells and stored as fat tissue instead of being burned as fuel. Researchers have also found that chylomicrons may play a role in the development of atherosclerotic plaque.

Medium-chain and short-chain fatty acids, however, go through a different pathway. After being absorbed in the small intestine, they travel directly to the liver via the hepatic portal vein. They can be absorbed into mitochondria, the energy producing units of the cell, without the presence of carnitine, a signaling molecule required for the absorption of long-chain fatty acids. There, they are preferentially metabolized for energy, usually resulting in high levels of acetyl CoA and the formation of ketone bodies. If you eat a particularly large amount of medium and short chain fatty acids in a meal, they will boost ketosis, even if the meal also contained a moderate amount of carbohydrate. In fact, without medium-chain fatty acids, it's difficult to restrict carbohydrates enough to consistently remain in ketosis. Ensuring that you include medium-chain fatty acids in your diet is key if you are following the modified ketogenic diet.

Coconut oil is the best whole food source of medium-chain fatty acids, containing about 63% (along with 30% long-chain saturated fatty acids and 7% unsaturated fatty acids). However, about three-quarters of these are the 12-carbon fatty acid lauric acid. Lauric acid is categorized as a medium-chain fatty acid because it does not require carnitine to be shuttled into the mitochondria and burned as energy, as do long-chain fatty acids. Our bodies don't process it like other medium-chain fatty acids, though, because only about 70% of lauric acid goes directly to the liver for fast energy release. The rest is circulated through the body like long-chain saturated fats. Thus, it's not quite as conducive to ketosis as 6-, 8-, and 10-carbon fatty acids are, but is nonetheless more ketogenic than other fats.

Butter, ghee, and other high-fat dairy products also provide a small quantity of MCTs, about 6% of total fat. This is usually not a major source of MCTs in the ketogenic diet, since these foods should be consumed in moderation due to their high long-chain saturated fatty acid content.

The best supplemental source of highly ketogenic 8- and 10-carbon medium-chain fatty acids is MCT oil, which is refined from regular coconut oil. With 8- and 10-carbon medium-chain fatty acids contents between 80 and 100%, it is the best way to deliver a major ketogenic fat boost to your diet. See the section on Supplements to Support Ketogenesis for more information on MCT oil and where to buy it.

Long-chain Monounsaturated Fats

Long-chain monounsaturated fats are a heart-healthy energy source and for many people, a major component of the ketogenic diet. While they are not as ketogenic as medium-chain fatty acids, they are a good choice for supplying your additional energy needs. The best sources of monounsaturated fats are high-oleic sunflower, safflower, and canola oil; extra-virgin olive oil; almonds, hazelnuts, macadamia nuts and their oils; and avocados and their oil. Monounsaturated fats make up at least 64% of the fat in these foods, and saturated fats less than 15%. Among these fat sources, olive and avocado are some of the best due to their very low omega-6 content (more on omega-3 and 6 fatty acids below). Try to consume most of your monounsaturated fats from olive and avocado, with moderate amounts of other nuts and oils.

Omega-3 and Omega-6 fatty acids

Polyunsaturated long-chain fatty acids do not make up a major source of energy in most diets, but certain types are essential in small quantities. You've probably heard about omega-3s, the class of fats found in fish, shellfish, and flaxseed, and in smaller amounts in nuts and beans. They are essential for many cellular functions, and they reduce inflammation and the risk for a range of chronic diseases. Only one type of omega-3, alpha-linolenic acid (ALA), is technically essential because the other omega-3s can be synthesized from it. However, conversion rates are low so it's good to get all three omega-3 fatty acids by eating fish in addition to the flax, hemp, nuts, and other plant foods in which ALA is found. You only need about 0.5-1.0g of omega-3 fatty acids per day.

Omega-6 fatty acids are another type of long-chain polyunsaturated fatty acid. As with omega-3s, just one type, linoleic acid, is essential in small quantities because the human body can use it to synthesize the other necessary omega-6 fatty acids. These fats have important roles in metabolism, bone structure, and reproductive function. Linoleic acid is supplied by vegetable oils such as soy, corn, canola, safflower, sesame, and sunflower, as well as chicken, beef, pork, and eggs. Some types of omega-6 fatty acids promote inflammation in the body, raising the risk of cancer, heart disease, and diabetes. Research suggests that linoleic and gamma-linolenic acid, found primarily in plant sources, are not as inflammatory, while arachidonic acid, found primarily in red meat, poultry, eggs, and milk, has a stronger inflammatory effect. The current recommendation is to consume about 2-4g of omega-6 fatty acids per day.

Over the past few decades, omega-6 consumption has increased greatly in the Western diet, a fact which many scientists believe is partly to blame for higher rates of chronic disease. The underlying issue may be less to do with omega-6 content itself than with the ratio of anti-inflammatory omega-3s to inflammatory omega-6s. The current western diet has an omega-3:omega-6 ratio of between 1:14 to 1:25, but diets with extremely strong scientific support, such as the Mediterranean diet, have a ratio of about 1:1, and many doctors recommend a ratio of no more than 1:4. Hunter-gatherer diets also likely ranged from 1:4 to 4:1. Luckily, it's not too hard to restore a healthy omega-3:omega-6 ratio on the ketogenic diet. Here are some simple tips to help achieve it:

- Eat 2-3 servings of fatty cold water fish each week, especially mackerel, salmon, cod, herring, whitefish, and sardines. Take fish oil supplements if you don't eat much fish.
- Include 1-2 servings of ground flaxseeds or flax oil in smoothies.
- Leafy greens and cruciferous vegetables (spinach, kale, watercress, Brussels sprouts, etc.) contain small amounts of omega-3s – these are a key part of ketogenic diets anyway, so make sure you eat plenty!

- Limit how much you cook with sunflower, corn, cottonseed, peanut, and soy oils. While they are low in saturated fat, they are very high in omega-6s and very low in Omega-3s.
- If you eat meat and poultry, do not buy conventionally raised, which have lower 3:6 ratios. Look for grass-fed or pastured. Grass-fed lard and butter have good 3:6 ratios as well, but should be limited due to high saturated fat content.
- Use mostly olive oil and coconut oil for cooking, which are relatively low in omega-6 fatty acids.

Saturated fatty acids

Not all saturated fatty acids are 'bad.' In fact, all of the medium-chain fatty acids in coconut and MCT oil are saturated, but they don't have the same kind of negative health effects that other saturated fats do. When we're talking about saturated fat, we're really concerned about long-chain saturated fats from red meat and high-fat dairy. These are the kinds of fat linked with heart disease, atherosclerosis, and high cholesterol. More research is needed on exactly how much saturated fat is safe to include in a ketogenic diet, but a safe target is no more than 20% of total caloric intake.

Aim to have at least half of this be medium-chain fatty acids, which are saturated but don't carry the same heart disease risk. Just 1½ tablespoons of MCT oil provide 20g. This recommendation is based on weight-loss studies of the ketogenic diet, in which participants ate high-fat diets containing up to 20% of calories from saturated fat without adverse effects to HDL, LDL, or blood triglyceride levels. This means that for a 1,800 calorie diet, no more than 40 grams of saturated fat should be consumed, with at least 20g as MCTs. If you have a family history of heart or artery disease, you should seek further advice from your doctor.

Meat and dairy fats can still be a part of the ketogenic diet, but should be eaten in smaller quantities than other fat sources. Chicken fat is one of the best choices, with 30% saturated fatty acids. Lard from duck, geese, beef, and pork is quite high in saturated fats, with 40-50% saturated fatty acids. These fats should be used in moderation. Butter and ghee are even higher in saturated fat, with about 60% of total fats being saturated. Similarly, the percentage of saturated fat in high-fat dairy products like cheese, sour cream, and heavy cream is very high. These foods are rich and delicious additions to the ketogenic diet, but they should be consumed in moderation.

Trans fatty acids

The largest source of trans fatty acids in the American diet is hydrogenated and partially hydrogenated vegetable oils, found in many types of processed foods. Very small amounts occur naturally in some meat and dairy products, but in most cases this is not a significant source. Hydrogenated oils are popular in the food industry because they can improve the texture of processed foods and increase shelf life. However, they are strongly linked with heart disease, higher LDL cholesterol, and weight gain. They should be totally avoided. This is usually not too difficult since the ketogenic diet excludes most processed foods, but check the labels of products like margarine and shortening, which are likely to contain them.

Protein Sources for the Ketogenic Diet

Protein is an important part of the ketogenic diet, but it must be supplied by a combination of foods that don't supply too much carbohydrate or saturated fat along with it. Legumes such as lentils, beans, and chickpeas, for example, are a great source of protein and contain no cholesterol and almost no saturated fat. But, they are too high in carbohydrates to be a regular part of the ketogenic diet. On the other hand, beef, pork, and lamb supply highly digestible protein along with some healthy fats, but they are also high in saturated fat and cholesterol. In addition, grass-fed meats can be quite expensive and have a huge environmental footprint.

The good thing is that there are many other keto-friendly sources of protein, including chicken, turkey, fish, shellfish, eggs, some types of dairy, and low-carb protein powders. Pastured poultry and sustainably caught or raised fish (see list of sustainable fish species below) have much smaller environmental impacts than red meats, and much lower levels of saturated fat and cholesterol. In the case of fatty cold water fish like salmon and sardines, they are also a great source of heart-healthy fats. Eggs and high-fat dairy provide highly digestible protein and fat, but it's important to eat them in moderation since some of it is saturated fat.

It's also important to avoid dairy products that are high in carbohydrates. Milk contains lactose, a naturally occurring carbohydrate. Just one cup contains 13g, nearly a third of the daily carb limit for most people following the ketogenic diet. Sweetened yogurts, ice cream, and other dairy-based desserts contain far too much sugar to be acceptable. Stick with high-fat dairy products like cream, sour cream, crème fraîche, full-fat cheese, and butter, which are much lower in carbohydrates, and eat them in moderation.

Low-carb protein powders are a great option for getting healthy, plant-based protein without the carbohydrates. Pea protein, brown rice protein, hemp protein, and soy protein are common options. They can be mixed into smoothies or baked goods to balance out a meal. See the Supplements section for more information on low-carb protein powders and where to buy them.

Overall, aim to get most of your protein from pastured poultry, fatty fish, and low-carb vegetable proteins, with eggs and high-fat dairy a few times per week and red meats no more than a few times per month.

Choosing Seafood

We mentioned sea food as a great option for supplying protein and healthy fats, but not all fish species are sustainable. The populations of many types of fish have been reduced by 90% or more and are in danger of total collapse, and some fishing methods end up killing dolphins, sharks, and sea turtles, too. In particular, make sure you avoid bream, sea bass, Atlantic cod, eel, grenadier, grouper, Atlantic halibut, marlin, orange roughy, parrotfish, ray, redfish, shark, Atlantic salmon, sawfish, smelt, sole, dogfish, sturgeon caught at sea, and almost all types of tuna.

Shrimp, salmon, canned tuna, tilapia, and pollock are consistently the most popular types of sea food in America. These species can be harvested or farm-raised in responsible ways, though it's not always the case. Even for sustainable species, the massive demand puts pressure on wild stocks. Choosing other types of fish for which there is lower demand helps diversify the fishing industry and protect more vulnerable species.

With these considerations in mind, we've assembled a list of alternative, sustainable, low-mercury, domestically caught or raised species that are a great addition to the ketogenic diet. This list is based on National Resources Defense Council and Monterey Bay Aquarium Seafood Watch recommendations. An asterisk denotes species that are a good source of omega-3 fatty acids.

- Anchovies*
- Arctic char*
- Clams, farmed
- Crab, brown
- Crayfish
- Hake
- Pacific Halibut
- Herring*
- Mackerel*
- Mussel, farmed
- Oysters, farmed
- Squid
- Sardines*

- Scup
- Sturgeon, farmed
- Tilapia
- Turbot, farmed
- Rainbow trout*

When buying any type of sea food, look for U.S. caught or raised. Many foreign countries have poor environmental and sanitary regulations, and the U.S. Department of Agriculture inspects *less than 2%* of all imported sea food. In general, the United States has stronger environmental regulations and much stronger food safety and health laws than other countries.

Carbohydrate Foods for the Ketogenic Diet

Since the portion of the ketogenic diet made up by carbohydrate-based foods is so low, it's important to choose your carb sources with care. As we've discussed, you will need to avoid carb-rich foods almost completely, including all grains, potatoes, pseudo grains like quinoa, most fruits, starchy vegetables, and sugars (including table sugar, maple syrup, and honey). Theoretically, you could eat about 50 grams of wheat, potatoes, or sugar each day and still stay in ketosis. The problem with this is that you would then have used up your carb allowance while adding little to no fiber, vitamins, minerals, or antioxidants to your diet.

Instead, aim to supply most of your carbs with foods that also supply fiber and micronutrients: leafy green vegetables, colorful non-starchy vegetables, cruciferous vegetables, asparagus, onions, mushrooms, berries, avocados, nuts, and seeds. These foods have just a few grams of carbohydrates per serving, so you can include many over the course of the day and ensure that your diet is varied and healthy.

Beginning the Ketogenic Diet

What to do Before Starting

There are two main things to do before starting the ketogenic diet: check in with your doctor and begin reducing carbohydrate intake. As we've just discussed, the ketogenic diet is not appropriate for everyone. It's important to talk to your doctor before starting to address any underlying health issues that could be aggravated by a major dietary shift. In addition, your doctor can take baseline blood pressure, cholesterol, and serum triglyceride measurements. For unknown reasons, some people just don't react well to the ketogenic diet and end up with dangerously high levels of fat in their blood. In some cases, this is due to poor fat and carbohydrate choices; in other cases, it may be for individual genetic reasons. Taking baseline measurements and checking in again after the first few weeks can help ensure that you aren't endangering your health.

The other things to do before beginning is start cutting down on the amount of carbohydrates you eat. A good target is to cut down by about 50g of carbs per week, an amount equivalent to a can of soda or two slices of bread. If you normally eat 325g of carbohydrates every day, aim for 275g per day over the next week, then 225g for a week, then 175g, etc., until you reach the 100 to 75g range. This gives your body time to start adapting before you begin eating just 30-50g of carbs each day.

Side Effects

The ketogenic diet can result in a variety of side effects, including increased thirst, fatigue, dizziness, fruity-smelling breath, hunger, trouble sleeping, nausea, constipation, and diarrhea. Most of these will dissipate after the first few weeks. If they don't, or are severe, discontinue the diet and seek medical advice. If you experience serious symptoms like throwing up, trouble breathing, or fainting, seek medical attention right away.

There are several things you can do to help ease mild side effects. As we discussed above, start reducing your carbohydrate intake before beginning the diet, so your body has time to adjust. It's also important to drink lots of water, as being in ketosis can increase water excretion. If you become dehydrated, consider rehydrating with an electrolyte-enriched formula to resupply potassium, magnesium, and other ions. Including exogenous ketones and MCT oil can be extremely helpful by supplying ready-to-use ketones and supporting fast ketogenesis to ensure that your body has a steady new energy supply after the reduction of carbohydrate intake. See the Supplements section for more information.

Finally, you must eat lots of leafy green and other non-starchy vegetables. Repeat: *eat lots of vegetables*! Whole grains and legumes are great sources of fiber in a normal diet, but obviously can't provide much for the ketogenic diet. This means that in order to avoid constipation and maintain good digestive health, you need to eat lots of vegetables to reach the recommended fiber intake of 25-35 grams per day. Nuts, seeds, and occasional servings of berries are also good fiber sources.

Supplements to Support Ketogenesis

MCT Oil

A variety of supplements are available to help you get and stay in ketosis. One of the easiest to include in your diet is MCT oil, a special type of oil derived from coconut. MCT oil may help reduce calorie intake, increase energy production, and promote weight loss. In both human and animal studies, addition of MCT oil to meals resulted in higher post-meal energy production and expenditure, and other studies have shown that they may reduce weight gain and increase fat burning. A trial with college students found that including MCT oil with breakfast helps maintain a feeling of fullness for longer and results in lower calorie consumption at the next meal. For these reasons, many of our breakfast recipes are smoothies that include MCT oil.

MCT oil is particularly beneficial for the ketogenic diet because it is metabolized more quickly than other fats and promotes ketone formation. As we discussed in the section on types of fat for the ketogenic diet, medium-chain fatty acids are transported directly to the liver to be used for energy, rather than transported throughout the body and stored as adipose tissue. Studies have found that consuming MCT oil with breakfast, even with a meal high in carbohydrates, resulted in significant levels of blood ketones, whereas equal amounts of other oils had no impact on ketogenesis.

Many people experience some nausea and gastrointestinal symptoms when they first begin taking MCT oil. These symptoms dissipate over time, but you can reduce them by slowly adding the oil to your diet. Start by including ½ teaspoon in your diet twice a day, for example in a smoothie and in a salad dressing, mixed with other fat sources. Over time, you can increase your total MCT oil intake to 3-4 tablespoons per day.

MCT oil should not be heated to over 150°C/300°F, because it will oxidize and develop unpleasant flavors. Thus, it is best used in smoothies, salad dressings, and low-temperature baking (no more than 160°C/325°F). The recipes section includes many ideas for how to use MCT oil in meals.

You can buy MCT oil from *Bulletproof Nutrition*[1], *KetoSource*[2], *NOW Nutrition*[3], and *Quest Nutrition*[4]. KetoSource and Quest Nutrition also offer MCT Oil powder, which can be added to smoothies, coffee, and baked goods just like MCT oil. In addition, KetoSource sells other keto-friendly fats including ghee, macadamia nut oil, and cacao butter.

Exogenous Ketones

Exogenous ketones are simply ketones produced outside the body. They can be a helpful source of energy as you begin the ketogenic diet and may ease some of the side effects, since you will have eliminated most carbs from your diet before your body has totally adapted to producing ketones. *KetoSource*[2] offers several types of exogenous ketone supplements, including chocolate and orange flavored powders that can be mixed with smoothies and shakes.

Low-Carb Protein Powder

As we discussed in the section on Protein Sources for Ketogenic Diets, low-carb protein powders are convenient options for supplying this key macronutrient.

NOW Nutrition [5] has one of the best selections of flavored and unflavored protein powders from soy, pea, brown rice, egg white, casein, and whey, some with just 1g of carbs per serving. *Bulletproof* [6] sells whey and collagen proteins specially formulated for the ketogenic diet, and *Quest Nutrition* [7] offers tasty flavored powders, including salted caramel and strawberries and cream. *Lucky Vitamin* [8] offers a range of protein powders including soy, brown rice, whey, and pumpkin seed, and many that are sugar-free.

Most websites have nutrition information easily available with each product description. Double check that the protein powder has no more than 1-3 grams of carbohydrates per serving, and no added sugar or other carbohydrate ingredients.

Carnitine

Carnitine is a small molecule that is essential for long-chain fatty acids to be taken into the mitochondria and metabolized to release energy. It acts like a shuttle, combining with the fatty acid to allow its entry into the cell and then passing back across the membrane to transport another fatty acid. It is supplied by meat, milk, and eggs, and can be synthesized by the body from the amino acids lysine and methionine. While carnitine deficiency in a normal diet is very rare, ketogenic diets that are very high in long-chain fatty acids may require more carnitine, because much more fat is being shuttled into mitochondria. Carnitine deficiency would thus decrease ketogenesis by reducing the rate at which long-chain fatty acids could be transported into mitochondria for use as energy.

Some studies have found that about 20% of people on a strict ketogenic diet had low carnitine levels during early phases of the diet, but more normal levels later on. Other research found that being on a ketogenic diet did not affect carnitine levels. Ultimately, more research is needed on this subject.

Since small doses of carnitine don't appear to have many health risks, some people prefer to use this supplement while following the ketogenic diet to ensure that a carnitine deficiency does not interfere with ketogenesis. This is more of a concern if your diet is high in long-chain fatty acids, especially if your diet also does not include many animal products. If your diet is high in medium-chain fatty acids and includes meat, milk, and dairy products, chances are low that you will need supplements, as carnitine is not necessary for medium-chain fatty acids to enter the mitochondria and what is needed will likely be supplied in the diet.

Most doses are around 1-2g per day. If you have peripheral vascular disease, high blood pressure, liver or kidney disease, diabetes, or a history or seizures, talk with your doctor before beginning carnitine supplements.

Monitoring Ketone Levels

If you plan to follow the ketogenic diet long-term, it is a good idea to invest in a ketone meter. These small medical devices can be used at home so you can check your ketone levels without the help of a doctor. Similar to blood glucose meters, they work by taking a tiny blood sample. Look for the Precision Xtra or the Freestyle Neo.

If you don't like needles, you can also use a urine ketone meter. They aren't as accurate, but still give you a good idea of your blood ketone levels.

When testing for ketone levels, you'll want to be in the range of 0.5 to 3.0 mmol/L. Lower than that means you aren't really in ketosis. Higher than that is a major cause for concern, though it is extremely unlikely to happen as a result of the ketogenic diet. Ketoacidosis is a life-threatening condition characterized by blood ketone levels of 6 mmol/L or more, usually caused by starvation or uncontrolled diabetes. If you detect very high ketone levels, seek immediate medical attention.

5-Week Meal Plan

A Note on Ingredients

Coconut cream is made by simmering four parts coconut with one part water. It is thick and high in fat, while being relatively low in carbohydrates. Do not confuse this with cream of coconut, which is sweetened. You can also make coconut cream from coconut milk by letting it chill for a few hours and scooping the fat that rises to the top off the remaining liquid.

We avoid including artificial sweeteners in most recipes, though flavored protein powders generally contain them. It's up to you if you want to add small amounts of stevia or xylitol to your smoothie, or substitute flavored protein powders for plain and avoid them all together. Some experts argue that artificial sweeteners are a safe addition to diets that makes them more palatable and keeps them low in sugar; others believe that artificial sweeteners distort our sense of taste and interfere with appetite regulation and cravings. We recommend avoiding them for the most part so that your palate naturally adapts to a low-sugar diet, but it probably doesn't hurt to add a little bit to smoothies every so often.

Feel free to use nut milks in place of water in any of the smoothies for a creamier taste. We have provided most recipes and nutrition facts using water for simplicity, in case you don't have nut milk at home. Most types are low in calories and carbohydrates, and you can simply add those macronutrient totals to your daily count.

Protein powders are a great way to make a Keto smoothie into an easy, complete meal. Make sure you find a low-carb, sugar-free type. Flavored powders are an easy way to make smoothies tastier.

Mayonnaise can be a great addition to a Ketogenic diet, if it is made with olive or other healthy oils and no sugar. Try natural food stores and check labels at the store, or make your own. Recipe below.

Things to Have in the Fridge/Pantry

Healthy oils and fat sources: olive oil, coconut oil, coconut cream, avocados, avocado oil, nuts and seeds (including almonds, walnuts, cashews, pecans, hazelnuts, Macadamia nuts, pumpkin seeds, flaxseed and flax oil, hemp seeds, sesame seeds, sunflower seeds), MCT oil, duck or chicken fat, beef or pork lard (use sparingly)

Non-starchy vegetables: dark leafy greens, tomatoes, cucumber, peppers, zucchini, onion, leeks, carrots, broccoli, cauliflower, kale, mushrooms, snap peas

Dairy: butter, ghee, heavy cream, sour cream, crème fraîche, cheese, cream cheese

Vegetable protein: Soy protein isolate, pea protein, brown rice protein

Animal protein: Fish, chicken, turkey, eggs; buy beef, lamb, and pork less often

Low-carb fruits: Strawberries, blueberries, raspberries, blackberries, watermelon

Keto-friendly sauces and condiments: mustard, vinegar, spices, herbs, salt, homemade mayonnaise, homemade creamy dips, homemade cream sauces

Day 1: Breakfast: Strawberry Chocolate Smoothie

    Lunch: Classic Chicken Salad

    Optional Snack: Keto Trail Mix

    Dinner: Shrimp Fried 'Rice'

Day 2: Breakfast: Chocolate Hazelnut Smoothie

    Lunch: Olive, Feta, and Sundried Tomato Salad

    Optional Snack: Keto Chocolate Truffle

    Dinner: Beef Chili

Day 3: Breakfast: Strawberry Cheesecake Smoothie

    Lunch: Creamy Spinach Soup

    Optional Snack: Keto Trail Mix

    Dinner: Roasted Tomatoes Stuffed with Goat Cheese and Bacon

Day 4: Breakfast: Orange Creamsicle Smoothie

    Lunch: Keto Egg Salad

    Optional Snack: Keto Peanut Butter Cup

    Dinner: Extra Creamy Broccoli Cheddar Soup

Day 5: Breakfast: Mushroom, Cheese, and Spinach Omelet

    Lunch: Green Omega-3 Boost Smoothie

    Optional Snack: Keto Chocolate Truffle

    Dinner: Simple Roasted Veggies with Creamy Garlic Sauce

Day 6: Breakfast: Vanilla Chia Pudding

    Lunch: Quick Taco Salad

    Optional Snack: Kale Chips

    Dinner: Pan-Fried Salmon Burgers with Garlic Aïoli and Greens

Day 7: Breakfast: Blackberries Cashews with Crème Fraîche

      Lunch: Salmon Salad with Balsamic Dressing

      Optional Snack: Celery with Peanut Butter Dip

      Dinner: Pan-Fried Chicken with Mushroom Cream Sauce

Week 2

Day 1: Breakfast: Coconut Cheesecake Smoothie

      Lunch: Roasted Eggplant Salad

      Optional Snack: Coconut Chai Fat Bomb

      Dinner: Gazpacho with Manchego Crisps

Day 2: Breakfast: Rose and Pistachio Smoothie

      Lunch: Greek Chicken Salad

      Optional Snack: Keto Chocolate Truffle

      Dinner: Cheesy Cream of Cauliflower Soup

Day 3: Breakfast: Aztec Chocolate Smoothie

      Lunch: Broccoli Salad with Peanut Sauce

      Optional Snack: Coconut Chai Fat Bomb

      Dinner: Pan Fried Rainbow Trout with Lemon Butter Sauce

Day 4: Breakfast: Scrambled Eggs with Mushrooms and Brie

      Lunch: Super Creamy Coconut Avocado Smoothie

      Optional Snack: Keto Peanut Butter Cup

      Dinner: Chili Chicken Bake

Day 5: Breakfast: Green Omega-3 Boost Smoothie

      Lunch: Veggies with Cream Cheese Sriracha Dip

      Optional Snack: Blue Cheese and Strawberries

      Dinner: Lasagna with Zucchini Noodles and Ground Beef

Day 6: Breakfast: Keto Granola with Berries and Crème Fraîche

Lunch: Frittata with Turkey Sausage

Optional Snack: Kale Chips

Dinner: Baked Hake with Caramelized Onions and Cherry Tomatoes

Day 7: Breakfast: Chocolate Chia Pudding with Almonds

Lunch: Baked Eggs with Tomato Sauce

Optional Snack: Salami and Cheese Roll-ups

Dinner: Baked Brie with Strawberries and Salad

Week 3

Day 1: Breakfast: Pumpkin Spice Smoothie

Lunch: Keto Egg Salad

Optional Snack: Coconut Chai Fat Bomb

Dinner: Turkey Burgers with Sage

Day 2: Breakfast: Keto Piña Colada

Lunch: Classic Chicken Salad

Optional Snack: Keto Peanut Butter Cup

Dinner: Cheesy Squash 'Noodles' with Tomato Sauce

Day 3: Breakfast: Scrambled Eggs with Spinach and Feta

Lunch: Golden Coconut Smoothie

Optional Snack: Keto Chocolate Truffle

Dinner: Extra Creamy Broccoli Cheddar Soup

Day 4: Breakfast: Chocolate Berry Avocado Smoothie

Lunch: Veggies with Blue Cheese Dip

Optional Snack: Salami and Cheese Roll-ups

Dinner: Pan-Fried Hake with Garlic Creamed Spinach

Day 5: Breakfast: Green Omega-3 Boost Smoothie

Lunch: Broccoli Salad with Peanut Sauce

Optional Snack: Coconut Chai Fat Bomb

Dinner: Cauliflower 'Mac' & Cheese

Day 6: Breakfast: Coconut Macadamia Chia Pudding

Lunch: Garlic Parmesan Mashed Cauliflower

Optional Snack: Keto Chocolate Pudding

Dinner: Baked Arctic Char with Sour Cream and Chives

Day 7: Breakfast: Keto Cereal with Berries and Cream

Lunch: Baked Eggs with Cheese

Optional Snack: Kale Chips

Dinner: Everything Burgers

Week 4

Day 1: Breakfast: Keto Chocolate Milkshake

Lunch: Roasted Eggplant Salad

Optional Snack: Keto Trail Mix

Dinner: Chilled Summer Soup with Asiago Croutons

Day 2: Breakfast: Lemon Meringue Pie Smoothie

Lunch: Watermelon, Mint, and Feta Salad

Optional Snack: Keto Chocolate Truffle

Dinner: Coconut and Almond Crusted Tilapia

Day 3: Breakfast: Scrambled Eggs with Avocado, Turkey Bacon, and Sour Cream

Lunch: Strawberry Chocolate Smoothie

Optional Snack: Coconut Chai Fat Bomb

Dinner: Italian Sausage with Sautéed Peppers

Day 4: Breakfast: Coconut Chai Smoothie

Lunch: Quick Taco Salad

Optional Snack: Keto Trail Mix

Dinner: Cheesy Squash 'Noodles' with Tomato Sauce

Day 5: Breakfast: Green Omega-3 Boost Smoothie

Lunch: Greek Chicken Salad

Optional Snack: Salami Cheese Roll-ups

Dinner: Broiled Rainbow Trout with Creamy Lemon Avocado Sauce

Day 6: Breakfast: Coconut Porridge

Lunch: Steak Salad with Blue Cheese Dressing

Optional Snack: Keto Chocolate Pudding

Dinner: Cheesy Cream of Cauliflower Soup

Day 7: Breakfast: Chocolate Chia Pudding with Almonds

Lunch: Creamy Spinach Soup

Optional Snack: Keto Trail Mix

Dinner: Chicken Stir-Fry with Peanut Sauce

Week 5

Day 1: Breakfast: Raspberry Macadamia Smoothie

Lunch: Keto Egg Salad

Optional Snack: Keto Peanut Butter Cup

Dinner: Pan-Fried Arctic Char with Creamy Avocado Herb Dressing

Day 2: Breakfast: Turtle Cheesecake Smoothie

Lunch: Classic Chicken Salad

Optional Snack: Keto Trail Mix

Dinner: Simple Roasted Veggies with Creamy Garlic Sauce

Day 3: Breakfast: Anti-Inflammatory Spice Smoothie

    Lunch: Mini Cream Cheese and Salmon 'Sandwiches'

    Optional Snack: Blue Cheese and Strawberries

    Dinner: Pan-Fried Chicken with Mushroom Cream Sauce

Day 4: Breakfast: Scrambled Eggs with Spinach and Feta

    Lunch: Chocolate Coconut Crunch Smoothie

    Optional Snack: Keto Chocolate Truffle

    Dinner: Poached Pacific Halibut with Lemon Herb Butter

Day 5: Breakfast: Green Omega-3 Boost Smoothie

    Lunch: Veggies with Cream Cheese Sriracha Dip

    Optional Snack: Coconut Chai Fat Bomb

    Dinner: Coconut Fish Curry

Day 6: Breakfast: Blackberries and Cashews with Crème Fraîche

    Lunch: Broccoli Salad with Peanut Sauce

    Optional Snack: Kale Chips

    Dinner: Keto Irish Beef Stew

Day 7: Breakfast: Pumpkin Spice Chia Pudding

    Lunch: Frittata with Turkey Sausage

    Optional Snack: Keto Chocolate Pudding

    Dinner: Cauliflower 'Mac' & Cheese

Keto Recipes

Smoothies, Pudding, and More

Fat Bomb Smoothies

Strawberry Chocolate Smoothie

Serves: 1

Total time: 5 minutes

Ingredients

- 1 tbsp. cocoa powder
- ½ cup strawberries
- 1 tbsp. coconut or MCT oil
- ¼ cup heavy cream
- 2 tbsp. low-carb chocolate protein powder
- water

Instructions

1. Blend all ingredients until smooth.

Nutrition Information

Total calories: 423; Calories from fat: 322

Total fat: 36.9g; Saturated fat: 25.9g

Total carbohydrates: 16.5g; Fiber: 4.1g; Net carbohydrates: 12.4g

Protein: 14.0g

Chocolate Hazelnut Smoothie

Serves: 1

Total time: 5 minutes

Ingredients

- 1 tbsp. cocoa powder
- ¼ cup hazelnuts
- ⅓ cup heavy cream
- 2 tbsp. low-carb chocolate protein powder
- 1 tbsp. MCT oil
- water

Instructions

1. Blend all ingredients until smooth.

Nutrition Information

Total calories: 571; Calories from fat: 475

Total fat: 54.7g; Saturated fat: 29.4g

Total carbohydrates: 10.7g; Fiber: 5.0g; Net carbohydrates: 5.7g

Protein: 17.7g

Serves: 1

Total time: 5 minutes

Ingredients

- 2 tbsp. cocoa powder
- 1 avocado
- 2 tbsp. low-carb chocolate protein powder
- ½ tsp. cinnamon
- pinch chili powder
- 4 tsp. MCT oil
- water

Instructions

1. Blend all ingredients until smooth.

Nutrition Information

Total calories: 501; Calories from fat: 351

Total fat: 41.8g; Saturated fat: 22.3g

Total carbohydrates: 19.9g; Fiber: 14.3g; Net carbohydrates: 5.6g

Protein: 27.3g

Chocolate Berry Avocado Smoothie

Serves: 1

Total time: 5 minutes

Ingredients

- 1 tbsp. cocoa powder
- ½ cup berries
- 1 avocado
- ¼ cup heavy cream
- 2 tbsp. low-carb chocolate protein powder
- water

Instructions

1. Blend all ingredients until smooth.

Nutrition Information

Total calories: 533; Calories from fat: 381

Total fat: 44.4g; Saturated fat: 17.1g

Total carbohydrates: 28.2g; Fiber: 13.4g; Net carbohydrates: 14.8g

Protein: 16.7g

Golden Coconut Smoothie

Serves: 1

Total time: 5 minutes

Ingredients

- ⅓ cup coconut cream
- 2 tbsp. low-carb plain or vanilla protein powder
- 1 tbsp. MCT oil
- 1 tbsp. ground golden flax seeds
- ½ tsp. turmeric
- water

Instructions

1. Blend all ingredients until smooth.

Nutrition Information

Total calories: 511; Calories from fat: 380

Total fat: 45.4g; Saturated fat: 38.7g

Total carbohydrates: 9.3g; Fiber: 5.2g; Net carbohydrates: 4.1g

Protein: 26.7g

Green Omega-3 Boost Smoothie

Serves: 1

Total time: 5 minutes

Ingredients

- ½ avocado
- 2 cups fresh spinach
- 2 tbsp. low-carb vanilla protein powder
- 1 tbsp. MCT oil
- 1 tbsp. flaxseed oil
- 1 tbsp. ground golden flax seeds
- water

Instructions

1. Blend all ingredients until smooth.

Nutrition Information

Total calories: 496; Calories from fat: 359

Total fat: 42.1g; Saturated fat: 17.1g

Total carbohydrates: 12.1g; Fiber: 9.4g; Net carbohydrates: 2.7g

Protein: 26.9g

Coconut Chai Smoothie

Serves: 1

Total time: 5 minutes

Ingredients

- ⅓ cup coconut cream
- 2 tbsp. low-carb plain or vanilla protein powder
- 1 tbsp. MCT oil
- ¼ tsp. each cinnamon and ginger
- pinch cardamom and/or nutmeg
- dash vanilla extract
- ½ cup strong black tea, chilled

Instructions

1. Blend all ingredients until smooth. Add water to reach desired consistency.

Nutrition Information

Total calories: 474; Calories from fat: 355

Total fat: 42.4g; Saturated fat: 38.5g

Total carbohydrates: 7.3g; Fiber: 3.3g; Net carbohydrates: 4.0g

Protein: 25.5g

Anti-Inflammatory Spice Smoothie

Serves: 1

Total time: 5 minutes

Ingredients

- 1 avocado
- 2 tbsp. low-carb plain or vanilla protein powder
- ½ cup blueberries
- 1 tbsp. MCT oil
- 1 tbsp. flaxseed oil
- ¼ tsp. each turmeric, ginger, and cinnamon
- water

Instructions

1. Blend all ingredients until smooth.

Nutrition Information

Total calories: 601; Calories from fat: 422

Total fat: 49.7g; Saturated fat: 18.3g

Total carbohydrates: 24.5g; Fiber: 12.6g; Net carbohydrates: 11.9g

Protein: 25.8g

Orange Creamsicle Smoothie

Serves: 1

Total time: 15 minutes

Ingredients

- ½ avocado
- ¼ cup heavy cream
- 2 tbsp. low-carb vanilla or orange cream protein powder
- ¼ - ½ tsp. orange zest, minced
- 1 tbsp. MCT oil
- water

Instructions

1. Blend all ingredients until smooth.

Nutrition Information

Total calories: 531; Calories from fat: 407

Total fat: 47.4g; Saturated fat: 29.3g

Total carbohydrates: 9.6g; Fiber: 6.2g; Net carbohydrates: 3.4g

Protein: 25.1g

Chocolate Coconut Crunch Smoothie

Serves: 1

Total time: 5 minutes

Ingredients
- 1 avocado
- 2 tbsp. low-carb chocolate protein powder
- 1 tbsp. MCT oil
- water
- 2 tbsp. chopped almonds
- 2 tbsp. unsweetened coconut flakes

Instructions
1. Blend the avocado, protein powder, MCT oil, and water until smooth. Stir in the almonds and coconut flakes and serve.

Nutrition Information

Total calories: 633; Calories from fat: 447

Total fat: 53.3g; Saturated fat: 24.9g

Total carbohydrates: 23.2g; Fiber: 16.3g; Net carbohydrates: 6.9g

Protein: 31.0g

Rose and Pistachio Smoothie

Serves: 1

Total time: 5 minutes

Ingredients

- ⅓ cup coconut cream
- 2 tbsp. low-carb plain or vanilla protein powder
- 1 tbsp. MCT oil
- 3 tbsp. chopped pistachios
- 1-2 tsp. culinary rosewater
- water

Instructions

1. Blend all ingredients until smooth.

Nutrition Information

Total calories: 554; Calories from fat: 396

Total fat: 47.2g; Saturated fat: 34.0g

Total carbohydrates: 13.3g; Fiber: 5.5g; Net carbohydrates: 7.8g

Protein: 30.1g

Lemon Meringue Pie Smoothie

Serves: 1

Total time: 15 minutes

Ingredients

- ¼ cup coconut cream
- ¼ - ½ tsp. lemon zest, minced
- 2 tsp. lemon juice
- 1 tbsp. MCT oil
- water
- ¼ cup plain homemade whipped cream
- 2 tbsp. crushed toasted cashews

Instructions

1. Blend first five ingredients until smooth. Top with whipped cream and toasted cashews.

Nutrition Information

Total calories: 519; Calories from fat: 456

Total fat: 53.8g; Saturated fat: 40.9g

Total carbohydrates: 11.0g; Fiber: 1.9g; Net carbohydrates: 9.1g

Protein: 5.4g

Pumpkin Spice Smoothie

Serves: 1

Total time: 5 minutes

Ingredients

- ¼ cup pumpkin puree
- 2 tbsp. low-carb vanilla protein powder
- 2 tbsp. MCT oil
- ¼ cup toasted cashews
- ½ tsp. cinnamon and ginger + pinch cloves or allspice
- water

Instructions

1. Blend all ingredients until smooth.

Nutrition Information

Total calories: 522; Calories from fat: 243

Total fat: 42.8g; Saturated fat: 29.9g

Total carbohydrates: 15.6g; Fiber: 6.5g; Net carbohydrates: 9.1g

Protein: 29.6g

Turtle Cheesecake Smoothie

Serves: 1

Total time: 5 minutes

Ingredients

- 2 oz. cream cheese
- 1 tbsp. MCT oil
- 1 tbsp. low-carb vanilla protein powder
- 1 tbsp. sugar-free caramel syrup
- water
- 3 tbsp. chopped pecans
- 1 tbsp. sugar-free chocolate syrup

Instructions

1. Blend the first five ingredients until smooth. Pour into a glass and top with sugar-free chocolate syrup and pecans.

Nutrition Information

Total calories: 498; Calories from fat: 419

Total fat: 49.1g; Saturated fat: 26.2g

Total carbohydrates: 5.8g; Fiber: 2.5g; Net carbohydrates: 3.3g

Protein: 12.8g

Strawberry Cheesecake Smoothie

Serves: 1

Total time: 5 minutes

Ingredients
- 2 oz. cream cheese
- 1 tbsp. MCT oil
- 2 tbsp. low-carb vanilla protein powder
- ½ cup strawberries, halved
- water

Instructions
1. Blend all ingredients until smooth.

Nutrition Information

Total calories: 514; Calories from fat: 411

Total fat: 48.0g; Saturated fat: 38.9g

Total carbohydrates: 9.5g; Fiber: 2.6g; Net carbohydrates: 6.9g

Protein: 18.7g

Coconut Cheesecake Smoothie

Serves: 1

Total time: 5 minutes

Ingredients

- 2 oz. cream cheese
- ¼ cup coconut cream
- 2 tbsp. low-carb vanilla protein powder
- 3 tbsp. unsweetened toasted coconut flakes
- water

Instructions

1. Blend all ingredients until smooth.

Nutrition Information

Total calories: 544; Calories from fat: 424

Total fat: 49.6g; Saturated fat: 37.3g

Total carbohydrates: 10.9g; Fiber: 4.6g; Net carbohydrates: 6.3g

Protein: 21.4g

Keto Chocolate Milkshake

Serves: 1

Total time: 5 minutes

Ingredients

- 1 avocado
- ¼ cup heavy cream
- 1 tbsp. MCT oil
- 1 tbsp. cocoa powder
- 2 tbsp. low-carb chocolate protein powder
- ½ cup water
- 3 ice cubes

Instructions

1. Blend all ingredients until smooth, adding more water as needed.

Nutrition Information

Total calories: 624; Calories from fat: 498

Total fat: 58.36g; Saturated fat: 31.1g

Total carbohydrates: 17.8g; Fiber: 11.8g; Net carbohydrates: 6.0g

Protein: 19.7g

Super Creamy Coconut Avocado Smoothie

Serves: 1

Total time: 5 minutes

Ingredients

- 1 avocado
- ⅓ cup coconut cream
- 2 tbsp. low-carb vanilla protein powder
- water

Instructions

1. Blend all ingredients until smooth.

Nutrition Information

Total calories: 551; Calories from fat: 411

Total fat: 49.0g; Saturated fat: 27.3g

Total carbohydrates: 18.4g; Fiber: 12.0g; Net carbohydrates: 6.4g

Protein: 20.5g

Raspberry Macadamia Smoothie

Serves: 1

Total time: 5 minutes

Ingredients

- ½ cup raspberries
- ¼ cup heavy cream
- 2 tbsp. Macadamia nuts
- 1 tbsp. MCT oil
- 2 tbsp. low-carb vanilla protein powder
- water

Instructions

1. Blend all ingredients until smooth.

Nutrition Information

Total calories: 535; Calories from fat: 425

Total fat: 49.6g; Saturated fat: 29.8g

Total carbohydrates: 12.5g; Fiber: 6.4g; Net carbohydrates: 6.1g

Protein: 18.2g

Serves: 1

Total time: 5 minutes

Ingredients

- ⅓ cup coconut cream
- 1 tbsp. MCT oil
- ¼ cup fresh or canned pineapple, chopped
- sugar-free sweetener, optional

Instructions

1. Blend until smooth, adding more water as needed.

Nutrition Information

Total calories: 535; Calories from fat: 466

Total fat: 55.7g; Saturated fat: 50.9g

Total carbohydrates: 13.5g; Fiber: 3.2g; Net carbohydrates: 10.3g

Protein: 4.6g

Coconut Almond Porridge

Serves: 1

Total time: 15 minutes

Ingredients

- ½ cup shredded coconut
- 2 tbsp. ground almonds or almond flour
- ¾ cup almond milk
- ½ cup coconut cream
- 1 egg yolk
- ¼ cup slivered almonds

Instructions

1. Combine the coconut, almonds, and almond milk in a small pot. Bring to a simmer and cook for 5 minutes, adding more water if needed.
2. Whisk together the egg yolk and the coconut cream and add.
3. Cook gently just until the porridge thickens. Served topped with slivered almonds.

Nutrition Information

Total calories: 739; Calories from fat: 492

Total fat: 58.7g; Saturated fat: 30.7g

Total carbohydrates: 35.5g; Fiber: 8.0g; Net carbohydrates: 27.5g

Protein: 19.0g

Blackberries and Buttered Cashews with Crème Fraîche

Serves: 1

Total time: 10 minutes

Ingredients
- 2 tbsp. butter
- ¼ cup cashews, finely chopped
- ½ cup blackberries
- 3 oz. crème fraîche

Instructions
1. Melt the butter in a skillet and add the cashews. Cook until golden brown. Top the crème fraîche with cashews and blackberries.

Nutrition Information

Total calories: 593; Calories from fat: 522

Total fat: 60.4g; Saturated fat: 25.8g

Total carbohydrates: 14.1g; Fiber: 6.4g; Net carbohydrates: 7.7g

Protein: 5.6g

Keto Cereal with Berries

Serves: 1

Total time: 5 minutes

Ingredients
- ¼ cup toasted coconut flakes
- ¼ cup slivered almonds
- 2 tbsp. chopped hazelnuts
- ½ cup half and half
- ½ cup berries

Instructions
1. Stir together the coconut, almonds, and hazelnuts in a bowl. Pour the half and half over and top with berries.

Nutrition Information

Total calories: 625; Calories from fat: 500

Total fat: 59.0g; Saturated fat: 23.3g

Total carbohydrates: 23.3g; Fiber: 11.2g; Net carbohydrates: 12.1g

Protein: 10.0g

Keto Granola with Berries and Crème Fraîche

Serves: 1

Total time: 5 minutes

Ingredients

- ¼ cup toasted chopped nuts
- 2 tbsp. toasted coconut flakes
- ⅓ cup crème fraîche
- ½ cup berries

Instructions

1. Mix together the nuts and the coconut. Sprinkle over the crème fraîche and top with berries.

Nutrition Information

Total calories: 442; Calories from fat: 363

Total fat: 42.6g; Saturated fat: 16.2g

Total carbohydrates: 16.2g; Fiber: 8.1g; Net carbohydrates: 8.1g

Protein: 5.9g

Vanilla Chia Pudding

Serves: 1

Total time: 5 minutes + overnight

Ingredients

- ¼ cup chia seeds
- ¼ cup heavy cream
- ¾ cup water
- 1 tbsp. MCT oil
- a few drops vanilla extract
- sweetener, optional
- ½ cup strawberries

Instructions

1. Mix together the first six ingredients and allow to sit for 8-12 hours, shaking occasionally if possible. Serve with strawberries

Nutrition Information

Total calories: 526; Calories from fat: 407

Total fat: 47.4g; Saturated fat: 28.9g

Total carbohydrates: 23.5g; Fiber: 15.2g; Net carbohydrates: 8.3g

Protein: 7.4g

Serves: 1

Total time: 5 minutes + overnight

Ingredients
- 3 tbsp. chia seeds
- ¼ cup heavy cream
- ¾ cup water
- 1 tbsp. MCT oil
- 1 tbsp. cocoa powder
- sweetener, optional
- 2 tbsp. slivered almonds

Instructions
1. Mix together the first six ingredients and allow to sit for 8-12 hours, shaking occasionally if possible. Serve with slivered almonds.

Nutrition Information

Total calories: 577; Calories from fat: 465

Total fat: 54.5g; Saturated fat: 29.7g

Total carbohydrates: 20.6g; Fiber: 14.2g; Net carbohydrates: 6.4g

Protein: 10.6g

Coconut Macadamia Chia Pudding

Serves: 1

Total time: 5 minutes + overnight

Ingredients

- 3 tbsp. chia seeds
- ¼ cup coconut cream
- ¾ cup water
- 1 tbsp. MCT oil
- sweetener, optional
- 2 tbsp. macadamia nuts, chopped

Instructions

1. Mix together the first five ingredients and allow to sit for 8-12 hours, shaking occasionally if possible. Serve with macadamia nuts.

Nutrition Information

Total calories: 564; Calories from fat: 463

Total fat: 55.2g; Saturated fat: 35.2g

Total carbohydrates: 18.3g; Fiber: 13.1g; Net carbohydrates: 5.2g

Protein: 7.4g

Pumpkin Spice Chia Pudding

Serves: 1

Total time: 5 minutes + overnight

Ingredients

- 3 tbsp. chia seeds
- ¼ cup heavy cream
- ¾ cup water
- 1 tbsp. MCT oil
- 3 tbsp. pumpkin puree
- 1 tbsp. sugar-free caramel syrup, optional
- pinch each cinnamon, ginger, nutmeg, and cloves
- 2 tbsp. chopped toasted cashews

Instructions

1. Mix together the first seven ingredients and allow to sit for 8-12 hours, shaking occasionally if possible. Serve with toasted cashews.

Nutrition Information

Total calories: 557; Calories from fat: 441

Total fat: 51.5g; Saturated fat: 29.9g

Total carbohydrates: 21.7g; Fiber: 12.3g; Net carbohydrates: 9.4g

Protein: 8.5g

Condiments and Add-Ons

Homemade MCT Oil Mayonnaise

Serves: 8 approximately 2 tbsp. servings

Total time: 5 minutes

Ingredients
- ½ cup light olive oil
- ¼ cup MCT oil
- 1 egg yolk (from a pasteurized egg)
- ½ tsp. Dijon mustard
- pinch salt
- 2 tsp. vinegar or lemon juice

Instructions
1. Whisk together the egg yolk, mustard, salt, and vinegar or lemon juice and put in a blender.
2. With the blender running, drizzle in the oils. The mixture should blend and have a smooth, light consistency. If it does not emulsify, try adding another egg yolk.
3. Keep in the fridge for up to one week.

Nutrition Information

Total calories: 184; Calories from fat: 182

Total fat: 20.9g; Saturated fat: 8.9g

Total carbohydrates: 0.0g; Fiber: 0.0g; Net carbohydrates: 0.0g

Protein: <0.5g

Avocado Dressing

Serves: 2 generously

Total time: 5 minutes

Ingredients
- ½ avocado
- 2 tbsp. lemon juice
- 2 tbsp. olive oil
- 1 tbsp. MCT oil
- 2 tsp. Dijon mustard
- 1 clove garlic
- pinch salt and pepper

Instructions
1. Blend all ingredients until smooth, or mash avocado with a fork and whisk well.

Nutrition Information

Total calories: 240; Calories from fat: 224

Total fat: 25.9g; Saturated fat: 9.6g

Total carbohydrates: 3.9g; Fiber: 2.5g; Net carbohydrates: 1.4g

Protein: 0.9g

Creamy Avocado Herb Dressing

Serves: 2

Total time: 5 minutes

Ingredients

- ½ avocado
- 1 tbsp. white vinegar
- 1 tbsp. olive oil
- 1 tbsp. MCT oil
- a few leaves fresh basil, cilantro, or chives
- a pinch dried thyme, oregano, or tarragon
- 1 clove garlic

Instructions

1. Blend all ingredients until smooth, or mash avocado with a fork and whisk well.

Nutrition Information

Total calories: 177; Calories from fat: 162

Total fat: 19.0g; Saturated fat: 8.7g

Total carbohydrates: 2.9g; Fiber: 2.3g; Net carbohydrates: 0.6g

Protein: 0.7g

Parmesan Crisp (Crackers or Croutons)

Serves: 2

Total time: 20 minutes

Ingredients

- 1 cup parmesan cheese, grated

Instructions

1. Line a baking sheet with parchment paper and spread the cheese in an even layer. Bake for about 10 minutes until the edges are golden brown.
2. Allow to cool, then break into large pieces to use as crackers, or small pieces to use as croutons for soup or salad.

Nutrition Information

Total calories: 216; Calories from fat: 126

Total fat: 14.3g; Saturated fat: 8.6g

Total carbohydrates: 2.0g; Fiber: 0.0g; Net carbohydrates: 2.0g

Protein: 19.2g

Serves: 2

Total time: 5 minutes

Ingredients
- ¼ cup peanut butter
- 3 tbsp. warm water
- 1 tbsp. MCT oil
- 1 tbsp. toasted sesame oil
- 1 clove garlic, minced
- ½ tsp. soy sauce
- ½ tsp. powdered ginger

Instructions
1. Stir all ingredients together until smooth. Add more water if needed, 1 tsp. at a time.

Nutrition Information

Total calories: 307; Calories from fat: 253

Total fat: 29.9g; Saturated fat: 11.3g

Total carbohydrates: 6.5g; Fiber: 1.9g; Net carbohydrates: 4.6g

Protein: 8.1g

Quick and Portable Meals

Classic Chicken Salad

Serves: 1

Total time: 10 minutes

Ingredients
- 3 tbsp. homemade mayonnaise
- 1 tsp. mustard
- 1 tbsp. minced onion
- salt and pepper
- ½ cooked chicken breast, cut into bite-size pieces
- 1 stalk celery, chopped
- ¼ apple, chopped

Instructions
1. Mix together the mayonnaise, mustard, onion, salt, and pepper
2. In a bowl, combine the chicken, celery, and apple. Add dressing and mix well.

Nutrition Information

Total calories: 452; Calories from fat: 303

Total fat: 34.7g; Saturated fat: 14.2g

Total carbohydrates: 8.4g; Fiber: 2.1g; Net carbohydrates: 6.3g

Protein: 27.9g

Veggies with Blue Cheese Dip

Serves: 1

Total time: 10 minutes

Ingredients

- ¼ cup crumbled blue cheese
- 3 tbsp. homemade mayonnaise
- 2 tsp. MCT oil
- 1 tsp. lemon juice
- salt and pepper to taste
- 2 stalks celery
- 1 cup baby carrots
- ½ cup cherry tomatoes

Instructions

1. Mix together the first five ingredients until smooth. Serve with veggies.

Nutrition Information

Total calories: 555; Calories from fat: 432

Total fat: 49.9g; Saturated fat: 28.0g

Total carbohydrates: 21.4g; Fiber: 7.3g; Net carbohydrates: 14.1g

Protein: 10.7g

Greek Chicken Salad

Serves: 1

Total time: 10 minutes

Ingredients

- ½ cooked chicken breast, cut into bite-size pieces
- ¼ cup crumbled feta cheese
- ½ medium cucumber, peeled, seeded, and chopped
- ¼ cup pitted green olives
- ¼ cup cherry tomatoes, halved
- 3 tbsp. homemade mayonnaise
- 2 tbsp. minced onion

Instructions

1. Combine the chicken, feta, cucumber, olives, and tomatoes in a bowl. Add the mayonnaise and minced onions and mix well.

Nutrition Information

Total calories: 533; Calories from fat: 412

Total fat: 46.8g; Saturated fat: 11.5g

Total carbohydrates: 9.2g; Fiber: 2.3g; Net carbohydrates: 6.9g

Protein: 20.6g

Watermelon, Mint, and Feta Salad

Serves: 1

Total time: 10 minutes

Ingredients

- 1 cup watermelon, cut into bite-size cubes
- 1 medium cucumber, peeled, seeded, and chopped
- 4 oz. feta cheese, crumbled
- ⅓ cup walnuts
- 1 handful fresh mint leaves, chopped

Instructions

1. Gently mix all the ingredients together. Chill for 2 hours before serving.

Nutrition Information

Total calories: 459; Calories from fat: 320

Total fat: 37.3g; Saturated fat: 14.4g

Total carbohydrates: 18.2g; Fiber: 3.1g; Net carbohydrates: 15.1g

Protein: 17.7g

Salmon Salad with Rich Balsamic Dressing

Serves: 1

Total time: 10 minutes

Ingredients

- 2 tbsp. homemade mayonnaise
- 1 tsp. Dijon or whole grain mustard
- 2 tsp. balsamic vinegar
- salt and pepper to taste
- 3 cups spinach mix or baby kale
- 3 oz. cooked or smoked salmon, in bite-size pieces
- ¼ cup chopped toasted walnuts

Instructions

1. Whisk together the mayonnaise, mustard, vinegar, salt, and pepper.
2. Put the greens on a plate and top with the salmon and walnuts. Pour the dressing over and serve.

Nutrition Information

Total calories: 597; Calories from fat: 452

Total fat: 52.0g; Saturated fat: 7.3g

Total carbohydrates: 10.2g; Fiber: 4.1g; Net carbohydrates: 6.1g

Protein: 26.3g

Olive, Feta, and Sundried Tomato Salad

Serves: 1

Total time: 10 minutes

Ingredients
- ½ cup green olives
- ¼ cup crumbled feta
- ¼ cup sundried tomatoes in oil, chopped
- ½ cucumber, peeled, seeded, and chopped
- 1 tbsp. olive oil
- pinch dried thyme and oregano, optional

Instructions
1. Toss all ingredients together. Serve right away or chill.

Nutrition Information

Total calories: 375; Calories from fat: 296

Total fat: 34.2g; Saturated fat: 9.1g

Total carbohydrates: 13.1g; Fiber: 4.4g; Net carbohydrates: 8.7g

Protein: 8.1g

Creamy Spinach Soup

Serves: 4

Total time: 25 minutes

Ingredients

- 4 tbsp. olive oil
- 1 small onion, chopped
- 2 cloves garlic, minced
- 1½ lbs. spinach
- 1 cup shredded mozzarella cheese
- 1 cup heavy cream
- 3 cups chicken broth
- pinch nutmeg
- salt and pepper
- 6 hardboiled eggs, chopped

Instructions

1. Heat the olive oil in a soup pot. Add the onion and garlic, then cook until softened and fragrant.
2. Add the spinach and cook until bright green and wilted, 2-3 minutes.
3. Transfer to a food professor and add 1 cup of broth. Pulse a few times until the mixture is creamy with a few chunks, or puree longer for a very smooth soup.
4. Return the soup to the pot and add the rest of the broth. Bring to a simmer and add the cream and the mozzarella. Cook just until the cheese has melted.
5. Divide between bowls and serve with chopped hardboiled egg.

Nutrition Information

Total calories: 517; Calories from fat: 371

Total fat: 42.0g; Saturated fat: 20.7g

Total carbohydrates: 14.6g; Fiber: 5.2g; Net carbohydrates: 9.4g

Protein: 24.6g

Keto Egg Salad

Serves: 1

Total time: 10 minutes

Ingredients

- 3 hardboiled eggs, roughly chopped
- ½ stalk celery, finely chopped
- 3 tbsp. keto-friendly mayonnaise
- 1 tsp. whole-grain mustard
- 1 tbsp. pickle, minced

Instructions

1. Combine the chopped eggs and celery in a bowl.
2. Whisk together the mayonnaise, mustard, and pickle and pour over the eggs. Stir well and serve or chill.

Nutrition Information

Total calories: 514; Calories from fat: 417

Total fat: 47.4g; Saturated fat: 18.2g

Total carbohydrates: 3.0g; Fiber: 0.6g; Net carbohydrates: 2.4g

Protein: 19.7g

Veggies with Cream Cheese Sriracha Dip

Serves: 1

Total time: 5 minutes

Ingredients

- 2 oz. cream cheese, softened
- 3 tbsp. sour cream
- 1 tsp. Sriracha sauce
- 2 tsp. MCT oil
- 1 green onion, thinly sliced
- 3 stalks celery, cut into 4-inch pieces
- ½ cup baby carrots

Instructions

1. Mix together the cream cheese, sour cream, Sriracha sauce, MCT oil, and green onion. Serve, or make ahead for a quick and easy lunch.

Nutrition Information

Total calories: 384; Calories from fat: 309

Total fat: 35.5g; Saturated fat: 24.1g

Total carbohydrates: 14.9g; Fiber: 4.4g; Net carbohydrates: 10.5g

Protein: 5.1g

Mini Cream Cheese and Salmon 'Sandwiches'

Serves: 1

Total time: 10 minutes

Ingredients

- ½ medium cucumber, sliced
- 2 oz. cream cheese
- 3 oz. smoked or cured salmon

Instructions

1. Top each slice of cucumber with a bit of cream cheese and salmon. Eat as a quick lunch or serve as appetizers.

Nutrition Information

Total calories: 313; Calories from fat: 203

Total fat: 23.0g; Saturated fat: 11.6g

Total carbohydrates: 7.7g; Fiber: 0.8g; Net carbohydrates: 6.9g

Protein: 19.8g

Steak Salad with Blue Cheese Dressing

Serves: 1

Total time: 10 minutes

Ingredients
- 3 tbsp. homemade mayonnaise
- 2 tbsp. crumbled blue cheese
- 2 tsp. lemon juice
- 3 cups mixed greens
- 3 oz. New York Strip or skirt steak, thinly sliced
- ½ cup strawberries, thinly sliced

Instructions
1. Whisk together the mayo, cheese, and lemon juice.
2. Arrange the greens, steak, and strawberries on a plate and drizzle with the dressing.

Nutrition Information

Total calories: 582; Calories from fat: 462

Total fat: 53.1g; Saturated fat: 28.1g

Total carbohydrates: 9.6g; Fiber: 3.5g; Net carbohydrates: 3.1g

Protein: 20.8g

Quick Taco Salad

Serves: 1

Total time: 10-20 minutes

Ingredients

- ¼ head lettuce, roughly chopped
- ¼ lb. ground beef, browned, or 1 leftover hamburger, crumbled
- ¼ cup shredded cheddar cheese
- ½ tomato, chopped
- 1 sliced onion, minced
- 2 tbsp. black olives
- 2 tbsp. sour cream

Instructions

1. Put the lettuce in a bowl (or a separate Tupperware container if you are packing this for later).
2. Toss together the ground beef, cheese, tomato, onion, and olives. When ready to eat, put all the toppings on the lettuce and drizzle everything with sour cream.

Nutrition Information

Total calories: 424; Calories from fat: 263

Total fat: 29.7g; Saturated fat: 14.1g

Total carbohydrates: 10.5g; Fiber: 4.6g; Net carbohydrates: 5.9g

Protein: 30.3g

Garlic Parmesan Mashed Cauliflower

Serves: 2

Total time: 20 minutes

Ingredients
- 1 head cauliflower (6-7")
- 4 tbsp. butter
- ½ cup sour cream
- ¼ cup grated parmesan cheese
- 1 clove garlic, minced
- salt and pepper

Instructions
1. Cut the cauliflower into large chunks. Boil or steam until tender.
2. Transfer to a food processor and add the butter, sour cream, garlic, cheese, and salt and pepper to taste. Process until smooth and serve.

Nutrition Information

Total calories: 470; Calories from fat: 334

Total fat: 38.0g; Saturated fat: 23.2g

Total carbohydrates: 24.8g; Fiber: 10.6g; Net carbohydrates: 14.2g

Protein: 14.6g

Broccoli Salad with Peanut Sauce

Serves: 1

Total time: 15 minutes

Ingredients

- 2 cups broccoli florets
- 1 tbsp. coconut oil
- ½ recipe peanut sauce
- 1 tsp. toasted sesame seeds
- 1 green onion, thinly sliced

Instructions

1. Sauté the broccoli florets for 4-6 minutes until tender and bright green. Toss with the peanut sauce and sprinkle with sesame seeds and green onion. Serve right away or pack as a quick lunch.

Nutrition Information

Total calories: 656; Calories from fat: 403

Total fat: 47.3g; Saturated fat: 23.6g

Total carbohydrate: 30.3g; Fiber: 13.0g; Net carbohydrates: 17.3g

Protein: 16.5g

Roasted Eggplant Salad

Serves: 2

Total time: 1 hour

Ingredients

- 1 large eggplant, cut into 1" pieces
- 1 medium onion, thinly sliced
- 1 red pepper, cored and chopped
- 4 tbsp. olive oil
- 3 cloves garlic
- ½ cup pitted green olives
- ½ tsp. each dried thyme and oregano

Instructions

1. Toss all ingredients together and roast at 400°F for 40-50 minutes, until the veggies are very soft and fragrant. Serve, or chill and pack for an easy lunch.

Nutrition Information

Total calories: 410; Calories from fat: 299

Total fat: 34.2g; Saturated fat: 4.7g

Total carbohydrates: 27.8g; Fiber: 13.1g; Net carbohydrates: 14.7g

Protein: 4.8g

Scrambled Eggs with Spinach and Feta

Serves: 1

Total time: 10 minutes

Ingredients

- 2 tbsp. olive oil
- 3 cups spinach
- 3 eggs
- ¼ cup crumbled feta

Instructions

1. Heat the olive oil in a frying pan over medium-low heat and add the spinach. Cook until wilted and bright green, 2-3 minutes.
2. Add the eggs and cook, stirring occasionally, until firm. Stir in the feta and serve.

Nutrition Information

Total calories: 591; Calories from fat: 455

Total fat: 51.2g; Saturated fat: 14.3g

Total carbohydrates: 6.5g; Fiber: 2.0g; Net carbohydrates: 4.5g

Protein: 26.8g

Mushroom, Cheese, and Spinach Omelet

Serves: 1

Total time: 15 minutes

Ingredients

- 2 tbsp. butter
- 1 cup button mushrooms, sliced
- 2 cups spinach
- 3 eggs, lightly beaten
- ¼ cup mozzarella

Instructions

1. Melt the butter in a skillet and add the mushrooms and spinach. Cook for 5-6 minutes, until soft. Season with salt and pepper and remove from pan.
2. Add the eggs and cook, without stirring, until they are almost cooked on top.
3. Add the mushrooms, spinach, and cheese and fold one half of the egg over on top. Continue cooking until the cheese is melted, flipping the omelet after a few minutes. Serve.

Nutrition Information

Total calories: 546; Calories from fat: 402

Total fat: 45.4g; Saturated fat: 23.0g

Total carbohydrates: 6.8g; Fiber: 2.0g; Net carbohydrates: 4.8g

Protein: 29.2g

Scrambled Eggs with Mushrooms and Brie

Serves: 1

Total time: 15 minutes

Ingredients

- 2 tbsp. butter
- 1 cup sliced button mushrooms
- 3 eggs
- 2 oz. brie, cut into small cubes

Instructions

1. Heat the butter in a frying pan over medium-low heat and add the mushrooms. Cook for 5-6 minutes, until softened.
2. Add the eggs and cook, stirring occasionally, until almost firm. Add the brie and cook for 1-2 minutes more. Serve.

Nutrition Information

Total calories: 636; Calories from fat: 481

Total fat: 54.4g; Saturated fat: 29.1g

Total carbohydrates: 4.2g; Fiber: 0.7g; Net carbohydrates: 3.5g

Protein: 32.9g

Scrambled Eggs with Avocado, Turkey Bacon, and Sour Cream

Serves: 1

Total time: 15 minutes

Ingredients

- 2 tbsp. butter
- 2 eggs, lightly beaten
- 2 oz. turkey bacon
- ½ avocado, sliced
- 2 tbsp. sour cream
- fresh chives or cilantro

Instructions

1. Melt the butter in a frying pan and add the eggs. Cook over low, stirring occasionally, until the eggs are tender and firm.
2. Microwave bacon for 4-7 minutes, until fully cooked and crispy.
3. Arrange eggs, bacon, and avocado on a plate. Top with sour cream and herbs.

Nutrition Information

Total calories: 638; Calories from fat: 505

Total fat: 57.5g; Saturated fat: 24.5g

Total carbohydrates: 8.8g; Fiber: 4.6g; Net carbohydrates: 4.2g

Protein: 24.1g

Sit-Down Meals

Mostly Vegetarian

Roasted Tomatoes Stuffed with Goat Cheese and Bacon

Serves: 2

Total time: 35 minutes

Ingredients
- 4 slices bacon, cooked and crumbled
- 4 oz. goat cheese, softened
- ¼ cup sour cream
- 1 clove garlic, minced
- 2 tbsp. grated parmesan or asiago
- 2 tsp. olive oil
- 4 large tomatoes

Instructions
1. Mix together the first five ingredients.
2. Cut the tops off the tomatoes and scoop out the flesh, leaving a hollow cavity. Brush on all sides with olive oil.
3. Divide the filling between the tomatoes and place on a baking sheet. Bake at 400°F for 20 minutes, until the tomatoes are softened and the filling is melty.

Nutrition Information

Total calories: 385; Calories from fat: 266

Total fat: 30.1g; Saturated fat: 15.1g

Total carbohydrates: 9.0g; Fiber: 2.0g; Net carbohydrates: 7.0g

Protein: 21.4g

Cheesy Squash 'Noodles' with Tomato Sauce

Serves: 4

Total time: 1 hour

Ingredients

- 4 cups squash from (approx.) 1 small spaghetti squash
- 4 tbsp. olive oil
- 1 onion, finely diced
- 1 pound 80% lean ground beef
- 3 tomatoes, chopped
- 2 tsp. Italian seasoning
- ½ cup grated parmesan
- 2 cups grated mozzarella

Instructions

1. Cut the squash in half and brush with oil. Bake at 425°F for 45 minutes.
2. Heat the olive oil in a large skillet and add the onion and ground beef. Cook for 10-15 minutes, until no pink remains.
3. Add the tomatoes and Italian seasoning, and bring to a simmer. Cook for 10 minutes.
4. When the squash is done, scrape the flesh into a large bowl. Add the sauce and parmesan and mix well to coat. Divide between four plates and top each with ½ cup mozzarella.

Nutrition Information

Total calories: 458; Calories from fat: 295

Total fat: 33.4g; Saturated fat: 12.7g

Total carbohydrates: 17.0g; Fiber: 3.4g; Net carbohydrates: 13.6g

Protein: 25.4g

Extra Creamy Broccoli Cheddar Soup

Serves: 4

Total time: 40 minutes

Ingredients
- 3 tbsp. butter
- 1 onion
- 2 cloves garlic
- 1 head broccoli, cut into small florets
- 4 cups chicken broth
- 2 cups shredded cheddar cheese
- 1 cup heavy cream
- salt and pepper to taste

Instructions
1. Heat the butter in a soup pot. Add the onions and garlic and cook until softened.
2. Add the broccoli and cook 5 minutes more, then add the broth. Bring to a simmer and cook for 15 minutes.
3. Add the cream and cheese, stirring well, and bring to a simmer again before serving.

Nutrition Information

Total calories: 554; Calories from fat: 441

Total fat: 50.2g; Saturated fat: 31.3g

Total carbohydrates: 9.6g; Fiber: 2.0g; Net carbohydrates: 7.6g

Protein: 19.2g

Serves: 4

Total time: 40 minutes

Ingredients
- 4 tbsp. butter
- 1 onion, chopped
- 3 cloves garlic, minced
- 1 medium head cauliflower, chopped
- 3 cups chicken broth
- 1 cup heavy cream
- 1 cup shredded mozzarella
- ½ cup grated asiago or parmesan

Instructions
1. Melt the butter in a large soup pot. Add the onion and sauté for 4-5 minutes.
2. Add the garlic and cauliflower and cook 3-4 minutes more, then add the broth and simmer until tender.
3. Transfer to a blender and blend until smooth. Return to pot, add cream, and bring to a simmer again. Stir in cheeses and serve.

Nutrition Information

Total calories: 508; Calories from fat: 386

Total fat: 43.9g; Saturated fat: 26.9g

Total carbohydrates: 14.8g; Fiber: 4.1g; Net carbohydrates: 10.7g

Protein: 17.4g

Gazpacho with Manchego Crisps

Serves: 2

Total time: 25 minutes

Ingredients

- 1 cup manchego cheese, shredded
- ½ cucumber, peeled, seeded, and chopped
- 2 tomatoes, chopped
- ¼ cup fruity olive oil
- 1 clove garlic
- ¼" slice red onion
- 2 tbsp. MCT oil
- handful fresh parsley and/or cilantro
- pinch salt and pepper
- ½ cup water

Instructions

1. Follow the directions for Parmesan Crisps, substituting manchego.
2. Meanwhile, blend the remaining ingredients until very smooth. Serve with manchego crisps as croutons.

Nutrition Information

Total calories: 587; Calories from fat: 503

Total fat: 57.7g; Saturated fat: 28.2g

Total carbohydrates: 7.0g; Fiber: 1.7g; Net carbohydrates: 5.3g

Protein: 14.1g

Baked Brie with Strawberries and Salad

Serves: 4

Total time: 45 minutes

Ingredients

- One 8 oz. wheel mild brie
- 2 tbsp. olive oil
- 1 tbsp. balsamic vinegar
- 1 tbsp. whole grain mustard
- salt and pepper
- 12 oz. arugula
- ½ cup toasted walnuts
- 1 cup strawberries, quartered
- 1 apple, thinly sliced

Instructions

1. Cut the top rind off the brie and place it on a small baking pan lined with parchment paper. Bake for 15 minutes at 350°F, until the cheese is soft and melty.
2. Meanwhile, whisk together the olive oil, vinegar, mustard, salt, and pepper and toss with the salad greens. Divide between four plates and top with the walnuts, strawberries, and apples.
3. When the brie is done, carefully transfer it to a cutting board. When it has cooled slightly, cut it and quickly scoop a quarter onto each plate.

Nutrition Information

Total calories: 404; Calories from fat: 281

Total fat: 32.5g; Saturated fat: 11.7g

Total carbohydrates: 15.4g; Fiber: 4.8g; Net carbohydrates: 10.6g

Protein: 16.8g

Chilled Summer Soup with Asiago Croutons

Serves: 2

Total time: 15 minutes

Ingredients

- 1 cup grated asiago
- ½ apple, peeled and chopped
- 2 cups loosely packed arugula
- 1 cucumber, peeled, seeded, and chopped
- 2 tbsp. olive oil
- 2 tbsp. MCT oil
- ¼" slice onion
- 1 clove garlic
- handful fresh parsley
- 1 cup water
- salt and pepper

Instructions

1. Follow the directions for Parmesan Crisps using the asiago.
2. Combine the remaining ingredients in a blender or food processor and blend until smooth. Chill, then serve with asiago croutons.

Nutrition Information

Total calories: 493; Calories from fat: 366

Total fat: 42.2g; Saturated fat: 24.6g

Total carbohydrates: 11.0g; Fiber: 1.7g; Net carbohydrates: 9.3g

Protein: 20.6g

Simple Roasted Veggies with Creamy Garlic Sauce

Serves: 2

Total time: 1 hour

Ingredients

- 2 cups cauliflower florets
- 1 onion, sliced
- 2 green peppers, sliced
- ½ cup baby carrots, sliced
- parsley, chopped, to taste
- salt and pepper
- 3 tbsp. olive oil
- 2 + 1 cloves garlic, minced
- ¼ cup sour cream
- 1 tbsp. MCT oil

Instructions

1. Toss the veggies with the olive oil, parsley, and 2 cloves minced garlic. Roast at 400°F for 30 minutes, until tender and fragrant.
2. Meanwhile, mix together the sour cream, MCT oil, and 1 clove minced garlic (or less, to taste). Serve the vegetables with the sour cream sauce.

Nutrition Information

Total calories: 386; Calories from fat: 283

Total fat: 33.4g; Saturated fat: 13.2g

Total carbohydrates: 22.0g; Fiber: 6.8g; Net carbohydrates: 15.2g

Protein: 4.8g

Cauliflower 'Mac' & Cheese

Serves: 2

Total time: 15 minutes

Ingredients

- 4 cups cauliflower florets, steamed
- 2 tbsp. olive oil
- 2 tbsp. minced onion
- 1 clove minced garlic
- ½ cup heavy cream
- ½ cup shredded cheddar
- ¼ cup grated asiago or parmesan
- 1 tsp. Dijon mustard

Instructions

1. Heat the olive oil in a small saucepan and add the onions and garlic. Cook for 2-3 minutes, then add the cream.
2. Bring the mixture to a simmer, then stir in the cheddar, asiago, and mustard. Cook over low heat until smooth and thickened. Add salt and pepper to taste, toss with cauliflower, and serve.

Nutrition Information

Total calories: 551; Calories from fat: 428

Total fat: 48.7g; Saturated fat: 23.7g

Total carbohydrates: 15.1g; Fiber: 5.2g; Net carbohydrates: 9.9g

Protein: 17.3g

Poached Eggs with Tomato Sauce

Serves: 2

Total time: 45 minutes

Ingredients

- 3 tbsp. coconut oil
- ½ onion
- 2 cloves garlic
- 3 tomatoes, chopped
- 6 eggs
- salt and pepper

Instructions

1. Heat the coconut oil in a frying pan. Add the onion and garlic and cook until soft. Add the tomatoes and continue cooking until it forms a sauce, 15-20 minutes.
2. Make a few spaces in the sauce with the back of a spoon and gently add the eggs to the skillet. Continue cooking, spooning the sauce over the eggs, until they are just set. Season with salt and pepper and serve.

Nutrition Information

Total calories: 445; Calories from fat: 321

Total fat: 36.5g; Saturated fat: 22.5g

Total carbohydrates: 9.5g; Fiber: 2.0g; Net carbohydrates: 7.5g

Protein: 21.1g

Baked Eggs with Cheese

Serves: 2

Total time: 20 minutes

Ingredients

- 2 tbsp. butter
- 4 tbsp. heavy cream
- 6 eggs
- ¼ cup asiago, grated
- ½ tsp. thyme
- salt and pepper

Instructions

1. Rub two small oven safe dishes (8 oz. or so) with 1 tbsp. butter each. Add 2 tbsp. cream to each dish.
2. Gently crack three eggs into each bowl and top each with 2 tbsp. grated cheese, thyme, salt, and pepper.
3. Bake the eggs for 12-15 minutes at 325°F until the yolks are just set.

Nutrition Information

Total calories: 479; Calories from fat: 366

Total fat: 41.2g; Saturated fat: 20.7g

Total carbohydrates: 2.9g; Fiber: 0.0g; Net carbohydrates: 2.9g

Protein: 23.5g

Turkey Burgers with Sage

Serves: 4

Total time: 40 minutes

Ingredients
- 1½ pounds ground turkey
- ½ small onion, minced
- 1 tsp. dried sage
- 1 egg
- salt and pepper
- 2 tbsp. butter

Instructions
1. Mix first five ingredients and form into four patties.
2. Heat a large skillet and add butter. Add the burgers and cook until well browned on the outside and no pink remains on the inside, 6-7 minutes per side. Serve.

Nutrition Information

Total calories: 326; Calories from fat: 189

Total fat: 21.1g; Saturated fat: 7.8g

Total carbohydrates: 1.0g; Fiber: 0.1g; Net carbohydrates: 0.9g

Protein: 31.4g

Pan-Fried Chicken with Mushroom Cream Sauce

Serves: 4

Total time: 25 minutes

Ingredients

- 2 tbsp. olive oil
- 2 chicken breasts, cut into bite-size pieces
- 2 tbsp. butter
- 3 cups button mushrooms, halved
- 1 small onion, finely chopped
- 2 cloves garlic, minced
- ¾ cup heavy cream
- ½ cup cream cheese
- salt and pepper

Instructions

1. Heat the olive oil in a large skillet. Add the chicken and cook until no pink remains, about 10 minutes.
2. Set the chicken aside and add the butter. Cook the mushrooms, onion, and garlic until soft.
3. Add the cream and cream cheese and stir until it reaches a smooth sauce consistency.
4. Add the chicken and heat thoroughly, then season with salt and pepper and serve.

Nutrition Information

Total calories: 523; Calories from fat: 371

Total fat: 42.1g; Saturated fat: 21.3g

Total carbohydrates: 5.8g; Fiber: 0.8g; Net carbohydrates: 5.0g

Protein: 31.2g

Chili Chicken Bake

Serves: 4

Total time: 1 hour including baking

Ingredients

- 2 tbsp. coconut oil
- 2 large mild green chilies, such as poblano, seeded and chopped
- 1 small onion, chopped
- 4 cloves garlic, minced
- 2 large tomatoes, chopped
- ½ cup canned chipotle chilies in adobo sauce
- Meat from 4 chicken thighs, cooked and chopped into bite-size pieces
- 2 cups shredded cheddar cheese
- 1 cup sour cream
- 1 handful fresh cilantro, roughly chopped

Instructions

1. Heat the coconut oil in a large pan. Cook the green chilies, onions, and garlic for 5 minutes, then add the tomatoes. Cook until very soft, about ten minutes.
2. Turn off the heat and stir in the chicken, chipotle peppers, and half the cheese.
3. Pour into a small casserole pan and top with the remaining cheese. Bake for 30 minutes at 350°F, until the cheese is melty and bubbling. Serve with sour cream and cilantro.

Nutrition Information

Total calories: 543; Calories from fat: 376

Total fat: 42.8g; Saturated fat: 26.0g

Total carbohydrates: 11.2g; Fiber: 2.5g; Net carbohydrates: 8.7g

Protein: 30.5g

Chicken Stir Fry with Peanut Sauce

Serves: 4

Total time: 25 minutes

Ingredients

- Meat from 4 chicken thighs, cut into bite-size pieces
- 2 tbsp. + ¼ cup peanut oil
- ½ cup peanut butter
- 3 tbsp. toasted sesame oil
- 2 tbsp. soy sauce
- 1 tbsp. lime juice
- 1 clove garlic, minced
- 1 tsp. powdered ginger
- 1-2 tsp. hot sauce, if desired
- 2 red bell peppers, chopped
- 2 tbsp. toasted sesame seeds
- 4 green onions, thinly sliced

Instructions

1. Heat 2 tbsp. peanut oil in a large frying pan. Add the chicken and cook for about 10 minutes, until no pink remains.
2. Meanwhile, mix together the peanut butter, ¼ cup peanut oil, sesame oil, soy sauce, lime juice, garlic, ginger, and hot sauce. Add more water if needed to achieve a smooth consistency.
3. When the chicken is done, add the red pepper and cook for 1 minute more.
4. Divide the chicken and peppers between four plates and top with peanut sauce, toasted sesame seeds, and green onions.

Nutrition Information

Total calories: 603; Calories from fat: 471

Total fat: 54.1g; Saturated fat: 10.1g

Total carbohydrates: 10.7g; Fiber: 3.5g; Net carbohydrates: 7.2g

Protein: 23.2g

Frittata with Turkey Sausage

Serves: 3

Total time: 25 minutes

Ingredients

- 2 tbsp. coconut oil
- ½ lb. ground turkey sausage
- ½ onion
- 2 cloves garlic, minced
- 2 cups small broccoli florets, steamed
- 2 oz. cream cheese, softened
- 6 eggs
- 1 cup shredded mozzarella

Instructions

1. Heat the coconut oil and add the turkey sausage, onions, and garlic. Cook until the turkey is thoroughly browned.
2. Add the broccoli, cream cheese, and six eggs. Stir well and continue cooking over low heat until the mixture starts to firm up.
3. Sprinkle the mozzarella over the top and transfer to the broiler. Cook for 3-4 more minutes until the eggs are firm and the cheese is bubbling. Serve.

Nutrition Information

Total calories: 567; Calories from fat: 363

Total fat: 41.0g; Saturated fat: 21.4g

Total carbohydrates: 12.5g; Fiber: 3.9g; Net carbohydrates: 8.6g

Protein: 37.9g

Seafood

Shrimp Fried 'Rice'

Serves: 4

Total time: 25 minutes

Ingredients
- 2 + 2 tbsp. coconut oil
- 3 cups grated cauliflower
- 2 bell peppers, chopped
- 6 green onions, thinly sliced
- 1 lb. shrimp
- 4 eggs, lightly beaten
- 1 tbsp. soy sauce
- 2 tbsp. toasted sesame oil

Instructions
1. Heat 2 tbsp. of coconut oil in a large skillet over high heat. Add shrimp and cook for 2-4 minutes until opaque and pink. Remove from pan and set aside.
2. Add 2 tbsp. coconut oil and add the cauliflower, peppers, and green onions. Sautee for 4-5 minutes, stirring frequently.
3. Add the eggs and soy sauce to the pan and stir continuously until the eggs are firm. Add the toasted sesame oil and stir, then toss with the shrimp and serve.

Nutrition Information

Total calories: 402; Calories from fat: 236

Total fat: 27.0g; Saturated fat: 14.6g

Total carbohydrates: 8.6g; Fiber: 3.5g; Net carbohydrates: 5.1g

Protein: 32.4g

Pan-Fried Salmon Burgers with Garlic Aïoli and Greens

Serves: 4

Total time: 30 minutes + 1 hour to chill

Ingredients

- 1 lb. boneless Pacific salmon filet, skin removed
- 2 eggs, lightly beaten
- pinch salt and pepper
- 2 tbsp. onion minced
- ½ cup homemade or keto-friendly mayonnaise
- 1 clove garlic, minced
- handful fresh cilantro, minced
- 2 tbsp. coconut oil
- 12 oz. greens, such as spinach, arugula, or mixed

Instructions

1. Finely chop the salmon with a sharp chef's knife into ⅛"- ¼" pieces. Mix with the egg, salt, pepper, and onion and form into four patties. Chill for 1 hour.
2. Meanwhile, whisk together the mayonnaise with the garlic and cilantro. Chill.
3. Heat the coconut oil in a large skillet and add the burgers. Cook for 2-3 minutes per side, until opaque throughout.
4. Serve on a bed of greens topped with the garlic aïoli.

Nutrition Information

Total calories: 523; Calories from fat: 387

Total fat: 44.0g; Saturated fat: 18.3g

Total carbohydrates: 3.4g; Fiber: 1.9g; Net carbohydrates: 1.5g

Protein: 29.9g

Pan Fried Rainbow Trout with Lemon Butter Sauce

Serves: 2

Total time: 25 minutes

Ingredients

- 1 tbsp. coconut oil
- 10 oz. rainbow trout filets
- 4 tbsp. butter
- 2 tsp. lemon juice
- 1 tsp. grated lemon zest
- salt and pepper
- 3 cups broccoli florets

Instructions

1. Heat the coconut oil in a large frying pan. Lay fish flesh side down and cook for 3-4 minutes until it starts to turn golden brown and releases easily. Gently flip each piece and cook for another 3-4 minutes until the flesh is opaque and flakes easily.
2. Meanwhile, steam the broccoli in the microwave or on the stovetop until bright green and tender.
3. In a small pan, melt the butter. Add the lemon juice, zest, salt, and pepper.
4. Remove the trout filets to plates and serve with the lemon butter and broccoli.

Nutrition Information

Total calories: 539; Calories from fat: 329

Total fat: 37.4g; Saturated fat: 21.1g

Total carbohydrates: 17.6g; Fiber: 7.8g; Net carbohydrates: 9.8g

Protein: 36.8g

Pan-Fried Hake with Garlic Creamed Spinach

Serves: 2

Total time: 20 minutes

Ingredients
- 10 oz. hake filets
- 1+ 1 tbsp. coconut oil
- ¼ onion, minced
- 2 cloves garlic
- 16 oz. spinach
- ⅓ cup heavy cream
- salt and pepper

Instructions
1. Heat 1 tbsp. coconut oil in a large frying pan. Add the hake, skin side down, and cook for 5-6 minutes. Flip and cook for another 3-4 minutes until the flesh is opaque throughout.
2. Meanwhile, heat 1 tbsp. coconut oil in a medium frying pan. Add the onions and garlic and cook for 2-3 minutes. Add the spinach and cook just until wilted.
3. Add the cream to the spinach and season with salt and pepper. Simmer for 2 minutes more until the cream thickens. Serve the hake with the spinach on the side.

Nutrition Information

Total calories: 425; Calories from fat: 260

Total fat: 29.9g; Saturated fat: 21.0g

Total carbohydrates: 10.7g; Fiber: 5.3g; Net carbohydrates: 5.4g

Protein: 32.4g

Baked Hake with Caramelized Onions and Cherry Tomatoes

Serves: 2

Total time: 25 minutes

Ingredients

- 2 onions, thinly sliced
- 2 + 2 tbsp. coconut oil, melted
- 10 oz. hake filets
- 1 cup cherry tomatoes
- salt and pepper

Instructions

1. In a large pan, heat 2 tbsp. coconut oil and add the onions. Cook over medium heat, stirring frequently, until they are golden brown and reduced greatly, about 30 minutes.
2. Meanwhile, lay the hake filets in a baking pan lined with parchment paper. Toss the cherry tomatoes with 2 tbsp. coconut oil and add them to the pan. Use a spoon to spread any excess oil onto the fish.
3. Bake the fish and tomatoes for 15-20 minutes at 350°F until the hake is opaque and flakes easily.
4. Serve with the caramelized onions.

Nutrition Information

Total calories: 404; Calories from fat: 243

Total fat: 28.2g; Saturated fat: 23.6g

Total carbohydrates: 12.8g; Fiber: 2.6g; Net carbohydrates: 10.2g

Protein: 4.8g

Coconut and Almond Crusted Tilapia

Serves: 2

Total time: 30 minutes

Ingredients

- 10 oz. tilapia filets
- ¼ cup ground almonds
- ¼ cup shredded coconut
- 2 tbsp. coconut oil, melted
- 1 clove garlic, minced
- 1 tsp. lime zest
- salt and pepper
- 1½ cups green beans
- 2 tbsp. slivered almonds
- 1 tbsp. butter

Instructions

1. Lay the tilapia on a baking sheet.
2. Mix the ground almonds, coconut, coconut oil, garlic, lime zest, salt, and pepper together and spread evenly over the fish.
3. Bake for 15-20 minutes at 350°F until the tilapia is opaque and the crust is crunchy.
4. Meanwhile, steam the green beans in the microwave or on the stove top until bright green. Toss with the butter and slivered almonds and serve with the tilapia.

Nutrition Information

Total calories: 560; Calories from fat: 362

Total fat: 42.3g; Saturated fat: 23.4g

Total carbohydrates: 14.6g; Fiber: 7.3g; Net carbohydrates: 7.3g

Protein: 36.5g

Broiled Rainbow Trout with Creamy Lemon Avocado Sauce

Serves: 2

Total time: 20 minutes

Ingredients

- 10 oz. rainbow trout filets
- 1 recipe <u>Avocado Dressing</u>
- 1 tsp. lemon zest
- 2 tbsp. butter, melted

Instructions

1. Pat the filets dry with paper towel and brush both sides with melted butter. Broil for 4-6 minutes until fish is opaque and flakes easily.
2. Meanwhile, make the avocado dressing, adding 1 tsp. lemon zest.
3. Serve the fish warm with the avocado sauce on the side.

Nutrition Information

Total calories: 531; Calories from fat: 381

Total fat: 43.6g; Saturated fat: 17.7g

Total carbohydrates: 4.0g; Fiber: 2.5g; Net carbohydrates: 1.5g

Protein: 32.0g

Baked Arctic Char with Sour Cream and Chives

Serves: 2

Total time: 25 minutes

Ingredients

- 10 oz. Arctic char filet
- 2 tbsp. mayonnaise
- ½ cup sour cream
- 3 tbsp. thinly sliced chives
- 2 cups steamed broccoli (serve on the side)

Instructions

1. Lay the Arctic char skin side down on a baking sheet. Use the back of a spoon to spread the mayonnaise over the top; this helps keep the fish moist while baking.
2. Bake at 400°F for 10-13 minutes, until the fish is opaque and flakes easily.
3. Serve fish topped with sour cream and chives and steamed broccoli on the side.

Nutrition Information

Total calories: 452; Calories from fat: 277

Total fat: 31.3g; Saturated fat: 9.7g

Total carbohydrates: 13.7g; Fiber: 5.2g; Net carbohydrates: 8.5g

Protein: 31.2g

Pan-Fried Arctic Char with Creamy Avocado Herb Dressing

Serves: 2

Total time: 20 minutes

Ingredients

- 10 oz. Arctic char
- 2 tbsp. coconut oil
- 1 recipe Creamy Avocado Herb Dressing

Instructions

1. Heat a large frying pan and add the coconut oil. Place the char filets flesh side down and cook for 4 minutes, then flip and cook for 4-5 more minutes until done. Serve with avocado dressing.

Nutrition Information

Total calories: 480; Calories from fat: 354

Total fat: 48.0g; Saturated fat: 21.6g

Total carbohydrates: 2.9g; Fiber: 2.3g; Net carbohydrates: 0.6g

Protein: 26.8g

Poached Pacific Halibut with Lemon Herb Butter

Serves: 2

Total time: 20 minutes

Ingredients

- 10 oz. Pacific halibut
- 4 cloves garlic, lightly crushed
- ½ cup dry white wine
- 2 bay leaves
- handful chopped fresh parsley
- 3 + 1 sprigs fresh thyme
- water
- grated zest of one lemon
- 4 tbsp. butter, softened
- salt and pepper

Instructions

1. Combine the garlic, wine, bay leaves, parsley, 3 sprigs thyme, and 3 cups water in a medium frying pan. Bring to a simmer and add the halibut. Add more water if necessary to cover the fish. Cook on low heat for about 10 minutes, until the fish is opaque and cooked through.
2. Meanwhile, mix the butter with the lemon zest and leaves from one sprig thyme.
3. Gently remove the fish from the poaching liquid and serve with lemon herb butter (poaching liquid can be discarded or used as soup broth).

Nutrition Information

Total calories: 346; Calories from fat: 227

Total fat: 25.7g; Saturated fat: 14.8g

Total carbohydrates: 0.0g; Fiber: 0.0g; Net carbohydrates: 0.0g

Protein: 27.7g

Coconut Fish Curry

Serves: 2

Total time: 20 minutes

Ingredients

- 1 tbsp. coconut oil
- ½ onion, chopped
- 1 red pepper, chopped
- 3 cloves garlic, minced
- ½ inch ginger, minced
- 1 15 oz. can coconut milk
- 2 tbsp. lime juice
- 1 tbsp. curry paste
- 8 oz. hake, in 4-5 pieces.
- handful fresh cilantro, roughly chopped

Instructions

1. Heat the coconut oil in a large pan and add the onions and red pepper. Cook for 3 minutes or so, then add the garlic and ginger and cook for 2-3 minutes.
2. Stir the coconut milk, lime juice, and curry paste together and pour into the pan. Bring to a simmer and add the hake. Cover and cook gently for 6-9 minutes, until the fish is opaque and flakes easily.
3. Ladle the curry into bowls and serve with fresh cilantro.

Nutrition Information

Total calories: 632; Calories from fat: 456

Total fat: 54.1g; Saturated fat: 45.8g

Total carbohydrates: 14.9g; Fiber: 1.8g; Net carbohydrates: 13.1g

Protein: 29.0g

Meat Dishes

Beef Chili

Serves: 4

Total time: 30 minutes prep + 2 hours simmering

Ingredients
- 2 + 2 tbsp. coconut oil
- 1 large onion, chopped
- 2 green peppers, seeded and chopped
- 3 cloves garlic, minced
- 12 oz. 80% lean ground beef
- 2 cups water
- 1 15 oz. can diced tomatoes
- 1 tbsp. cocoa powder
- 2 tsp. Worcestershire sauce
- 1 tsp. oregano
- 1-2 tsp. chili powder
- salt and pepper
- ½ cup sour cream
- ½ cup shredded cheddar cheese
- green onions, thinly sliced

Instructions
1. Heat 2 tbsp. coconut oil in a large skillet. Add the onions, peppers, and garlic and cook until softened.
2. Meanwhile, heat 2 tbsp. coconut oil in a soup pot. Add the ground beef and cook until browned.
3. Add the peppers, onions, tomatoes, water, cocoa powder, Worcestershire sauce oregano, chili powder, salt, and pepper to the pot with the beef. Simmer, covered, for about 2 hours. Add more water if needed.
4. Serve with cheese, sour cream, and green onions.

Nutrition Information

Total calories: 501; Calories from fat: 345

Total fat: 39.1g; Saturated fat: 23.7g

Total carbohydrates: 10.4g; Fiber: 2.8g; Net carbohydrates: 7.6g

Protein: 29.3g

Lasagna with Zucchini Noodles and Ground Beef

Serves: 6

Total time: 25 minutes prep + 30 minutes baking

Ingredients

- 4 medium zucchini, very thinly sliced lengthwise on a mandoline
- 1 tbsp. + 2 tbsp. olive oil
- 1 onion, finely chopped
- 3 cloves garlic, minced
- 1½ lbs. 80% lean ground beef
- 3 tomatoes, chopped
- ½ each dried thyme, oregano, and basil
- 3 cups shredded mozzarella
- 1 cup grated parmesan
- salt and pepper

Instructions

1. Heat a large frying pan and add 1 tbsp. olive oil. Cook the zucchini slices for 2 minutes per side, until softened. Allow to drain on paper towels, pressing gently to remove excess moisture.
2. Heat 2 tbsp. olive oil in the frying pan and add the onion and garlic. Cook until softened and fragrant, 6-7 minutes, then add the ground beef.
3. Brown thoroughly, then add the chopped tomato and herbs. Cook until the tomatoes have softened and formed a sauce, about 10 minutes. Add salt and pepper to taste.
4. Lay ⅓ of the zucchini slices in the bottom of a medium casserole dish. Spread ⅓ of the ground beef mixture over it and sprinkle with 1 cup mozzarella and ⅓ cup parmesan. Repeat this layering three times.
5. Bake for 20-30 minutes at 350°F until the cheese is melted and the sauce is bubbling.

Nutrition Information

Total calories: 645; Calories from fat: 392

Total fat: 44.1g; Saturated fat: 18.7g

Total carbohydrates: 9.8g; Fiber: 2.2g; Net carbohydrates: 7.6g

Protein: 51.9g

Italian Sausage with Sautéed Peppers

Serves: 4

Total time: 30 minutes

Ingredients
- 3 tbsp. olive oil
- 4 sweet bell peppers – mix of colors
- 1 onion
- 3 cloves garlic
- 2 tsp. Italian seasoning
- 2 lbs. sweet Italian sausage, sliced

Instructions
1. Heat the olive oil in a large pan and add the peppers, onion, and garlic. Cook for 4-5 minutes, until fragrant and tender. Add the Italian seasoning and remove from pan.
2. Add the sausage to the pan and cook thoroughly, 10-12 minutes. Return the peppers to the pan and mix everything together. Serve.

Nutrition Information

Total calories: 468; Calories from fat: 267

Total fat: 29.8g; Saturated fat: 9.0g

Total carbohydrates: 12.9g; Fiber: 2.5g; Net carbohydrates: 10.4g

Protein: 38.6g

Everything Burgers

Serves: 2

Total time: 30 minutes

Ingredients

- ½ lb. 80% lean ground beef
- 1 tsp. Worcestershire sauce
- 2 slices cheddar cheese
- 4 strips crispy bacon
- 2 slices red onion
- ½ head butter or Bibb lettuce
- 1 avocado, sliced
- 1 tomato, sliced
- 1 large dill pickle, sliced
- mustard to taste

Instructions

1. Mix the ground beef with the Worcestershire sauce and form into two patties. Grill or pan fry over medium until no pink remains in the center, 5-7 minutes per side.
2. When the burgers are almost done, lay a slice of cheese on top and allow to melt.
3. Divide the lettuce between two plates and set the burgers on top. Top with red onion, avocado, tomato, bacon, pickle, and mustard.

Nutrition Information

Total calories: 545; Calories from fat: 348

Total fat: 39.6g; Saturated fat: 14.5g

Total carbohydrates: 13.0g; Fiber: 7.4g; Net carbohydrates: 5.6g

Protein: 36.2g

Keto Irish Beef Stew

Serves: 4

Total time: 2 hours

Ingredients

- 3 tbsp. coconut oil
- 1 lb. high-fat beef stew meat, such as chuck, cut into 1" pieces
- 1 onion, chopped
- ¼ lb. carrots, chopped
- ¼ lb. parsnips, chopped
- 4 cloves garlic, chopped
- handful fresh parsley
- salt and pepper
- ½ tsp. thyme
- 2 bay leaves
- 2 tsp. Worcestershire sauce
- 1 cup Guinness stout
- 1 qt. beef broth

Instructions

1. Heat the coconut oil in a soup pot and add the beef. Brown, then add the rest of the ingredients.
2. Simmer for 1½ - 2 hours until the beef is tender and the broth is thickened, adding more water as needed.

Nutrition Information

Total calories: 496; Calories from fat: 285

Total fat: 32.0g; Saturated fat: 17.5g

Total carbohydrates: 12.9g; Fiber: 3.0g; Net carbohydrates: 9.9g

Protein: 36.0g

Snacks

Keto Chocolate Coconut Truffles

Serves: 16

Total time: 25 minutes

Ingredients
- 1-100g bar 85% dark chocolate, chopped
- ½ cup coconut oil
- 1 cup unsweetened shredded coconut
- ¼ cup cocoa powder
- sweetener, optional

Instructions
1. Melt the coconut oil over very low heat in a small saucepan. Add the chocolate and stir until smooth.
2. Add the coconut and sweetener and stir well.
3. Cool until firm enough to shape, then form into 12 balls and roll in the cocoa powder. Store in the fridge for up to two weeks or the freezer for up to two months.

Nutrition Information

Total calories: 133; Calories from fat: 116

Total fat: 13.2g; Saturated fat: 10.8g

Total carbohydrates: 4.4g; Fiber: 2.2g; Net carbohydrates: 2.2g

Protein: 1.4g

Serves: 1

Total time: 5 minutes

Ingredients

- 4 slices salami
- 4 slices mild cheddar cheese (totaling 1 oz.)

Instructions

1. Lay each slice of salami on a slice of cheese. Roll up and eat.

Nutrition Information

Total calories: 245; Calories from fat: 174

Total fat: 19.6g; Saturated fat: 9.9g

Total carbohydrates: 0.9g; Fiber: 0.0g; Net carbohydrates: 0.9g

Protein: 16.3g

Keto Peanut Butter Cups

Serves: 10

Total time: 20 minutes + chilling

Ingredients

- ¾ cup peanut butter
- ½ cup coconut oil
- sweetener, optional
- 1-100g bar 85% dark chocolate
- 3 tbsp. butter

Instructions

1. Line a muffin pan with 10 paper muffin cups.
2. Melt the coconut oil in the microwave or over a double boiler and mix with the peanut butter. Add the sweetener if using.
3. Put 2 tbsp. of the mixture in each paper cup.
4. Melt the dark chocolate and butter in the microwave (on very low power) or over a double boiler. Distribute a layer of chocolate evenly across the ten cups.
5. Put the cups in the fridge. Store for two weeks in the fridge or two months in the freezer.

Nutrition Information

Total calories: 196; Calories from fat: 177

Total fat: 20.0g; Saturated fat: 14.6g

Total carbohydrates: 4.2g; Fiber: 1.6g; Net carbohydrates: 2.6g

Protein: 1.9g

Blue Cheese and Strawberries

Serves: 1

Total time: 5 minutes

Ingredients
- 2 oz. blue cheese
- ½ cup strawberries

Instructions
1. Cut the strawberries lengthwise into thick slices. Thinly slice the blue cheese and eat each piece with a slice of strawberry.

Nutrition Information

Total calories: 222; Calories from fat: 143

Total fat: 16.3g; Saturated fat: 10.5g

Total carbohydrates: 7.1g; Fiber: 1.5g; Net carbohydrates: 5.6g

Protein: 12.5g

Coconut Chai Fat Bombs

Serves: 12

Total time: 25 minutes

Ingredients
- ½ cup coconut oil
- ¾ cup + ¼ cup unsweetened shredded coconut
- ½ tsp. cinnamon
- ½ tsp. ginger
- ½ tsp. cardamom
- ¼ tsp. nutmeg
- dash vanilla extract
- sweetener, optional

Instructions
1. Melt the coconut oil over very low heat in a small saucepan. Add ¾ cup coconut, spices, vanilla, and sweetener and stir well.
2. Cool until firm enough to shape, then form into 12 balls and roll in the remaining shredded coconut. Store in the fridge for up to two weeks or the freezer for up to two months.

Nutrition Information

Total calories: 126; Calories from fat: 117

Total fat: 13.7g; Saturated fat: 11.9g

Total carbohydrates: 2.0g; Fiber: 1.4g; Net carbohydrates: 0.6g

Protein: 0.5g

Keto Chocolate Pudding

Serves: 2

Total time: 5 minutes

Ingredients
- 1 avocado
- ½ cup heavy cream
- 3 tbsp. cocoa powder
- zero-calorie sweetener to taste

Instructions
1. Blend all ingredients in a blender or food processor until very smooth. You can add more cream if needed to adjust the texture.

Nutrition Information

Total calories: 337; Calories from fat: 290

Total fat: 33.5g; Saturated fat: 15.8g

Total carbohydrates: 12.1g; Fiber: 7.2g; Net carbohydrates: 4.9g

Protein: 4.1g

Total time: 5 minutes

Serves: 12 servings (¼ cup)

Ingredients

- 1 cup chopped macadamia nuts
- 1 cup toasted pumpkin seeds
- 1 3.5oz. bar sugar-free or 85% dark chocolate, broken into pieces
- ½ cup toasted unsweetened coconut flakes

Instruction

1. Mix all ingredients together and store in an airtight container.

Nutrition Information

Total calories: 176; Calories from fat: 130

Total fat: 15.2g; Saturated fat: 5.6g

Total carbohydrates: 9.0g; Fiber: 2.4g; Net carbohydrates: 6.6g

Protein: 2.7g

Celery with Peanut Butter Dip

Serves: 1

Total time: 5 minutes

Ingredients
- 2 tbsp. peanut butter (no sugar added)
- 2 tsp. MCT oil
- 2 large stalks celery, cut into 4-inch pieces

Instructions
1. Stir together the peanut butter and MCT oil until smooth. Serve with celery.

Nutrition Information

Total calories: 279; Calories from fat: 214

Total fat: 25.5g; Saturated fat: 12.6g

Total carbohydrates: 9.1g; Fiber: 3.2g; Net carbohydrates: 5.9g

Protein: 8.6g

Serves: 2

Total time: 35 minutes

Ingredients

- 4 cups kale, with large stems removed and leaves torn into large pieces
- 1 tbsp. coconut oil, melted
- 2 tbsp. finely grated parmesan
- salt and pepper
- pinch garlic and onion powder if desired

Instructions

1. Toss the kale pieces with the coconut oil and mix very well, using your hands to coat each piece thoroughly.
2. Toss with the parmesan cheese and spices. Spread in a single layer on a parchment-paper lined baking sheet (you may need to do several batches).
3. Bake at 320°F for 20-25 minutes, stirring gently halfway through, until the leaves are crispy. Cool completely, then store in an airtight container.

Nutrition Information

Total calories: 130; Calories from fat: 77

Total fat: 8.9g; Saturated fat: 6.8g

Total carbohydrates: 10.3g; Fiber: 2.0g; Net carbohydrates: 8.3g

Protein: 5.2g

Conclusion

We hope that you feel prepared to start the ketogenic diet after finishing this book. You now know who should try the ketogenic diet, what to do before starting, how to minimize side effects, what types of foods to eat, and how to supplement your diet with MCT oil and exogenous ketones. In addition, you have over ninety recipes to choose from over the next several weeks. We hope you'll enjoy using them as an introduction to ketogenic cooking and as inspiration for your own recipe ideas.

Now, it's time to get started! In the next few days, start cutting back on carb foods. Schedule an appointment with your doctor. Stock up on healthy fats and keto-friendly proteins, and order supplements from online retailers. After reading this book, you have the knowledge and resources to get started on a diet that could help you lose weight and improve your health – now it's up to you!

Best of luck and bon appétit!

And Please...

If you'd like more quality diet books at this low price, we'd really appreciate a review on Amazon. The number of reviews a book has is directly related to how it sells, so even leaving a very short review will help make it possible for us to continue to do what we do.

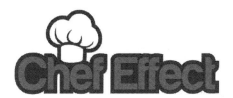

Sources

[1] http://www.bulletproof.com/nutrition/quality-fats/

[2] https://ketosource.co.uk/

[3] https://www.nowfoods.com/sports-nutrition/mct-oil-liquid

[4] http://www.questnutrition.com/protein-powders/mct-oil-powder/

[5] https://www.nowfoods.com/sports-nutrition/by-category/protein-powders

[6] http://www.bulletproof.com/nutrition/proteins/

[7] http://www.questnutrition.com/protein-powders

[8] https://www.luckyvitamin.com/

Other Books by Chef Effect

To find out more about other books that we have written, please visit our Author Central Page by going to the webpage below or scanning the QR code.

https://goo.gl/5IUi6k

Made in the USA
Lexington, KY
26 August 2017